Dental Bleaching

Dental Bleaching

By

Martin G D Kelleher

Editor-in-Chief: Nairn H F Wilson
Editor Operative Dentistry: Paul A Brunton

Quintessence Publishing Co. Ltd.
London, Berlin, Chicago, Paris, Milan, Barcelona, Istanbul,
São Paulo, Tokyo, New Delhi, Moscow, Prague, Warsaw

British Library Cataloguing in Publication Data

Kelleher, Martin
  Dental bleaching. - (Quintessentials of dental practice; v. 38)
  1. Teeth - Bleaching
  I. Title II. Wilson, Nairn H. F.
  617.6'34

ISBN: 9781850971313

ISBN: 978-1-85097-131-3

Foreword

Bleaching, although not new to dentistry, has recently become extremely popular. It has the great advantage of being minimally interventive and, assuming correct use, safe. In addition, the appropriate application of bleaching agents and techniques does not adversely affect the integrity or properties of sound tooth tissues.

As emphasised in this most attractive addition to the multidisciplinary *Quintessentials* series, practitioners and students must not be lulled into a false sense of complacency by the apparent simplicity and versatility of most bleaching techniques. Careful diagnosis, informed treatment planning, patient consent and cooperation and effective troubleshooting are all critical to predictable success and good, long-term clinical outcomes. Bleaching is best provided as part of the holistic care of patients seeking, together with other outcomes, an improvement in their dental attractiveness. While long-term outcomes of bleaching can be excellent, monitoring and "top-up" treatments may be required as part of longitudinal, patient-centred care.

Whatever your views on bleaching and your application of tooth lightening techniques in your clinical practice, this *Quintessentials* volume will be a great asset. It is succinct, authoritative, beautifully illustrated, affordable and, above all else, of immediate practical application and relevance. What more could the busy practitioner or student wish of a book? Pragmatism: well it has that too, and in abundance. For a fraction of the cost of a bleaching treatment, this *Quintessentials* volume is, in common with all its sibling volumes, quintessential value for money.

Bleaching is firmly established as an element of the modern clinical practice of dentistry, and practitioners and students must understand the mechanisms, application and pitfalls of the relevant techniques. This book meets these needs, and provides an opportunity to be one step closer to satisfying the ever-increasing expectations of patients.

Congratulations to the author on a job well done.

Nairn Wilson
Editor-in-Chief

Preface

Bleaching has been scientifically proven to be safe and very effective in altering the colour of teeth. Discoloured teeth are up to five times more worrying to patients than crooked teeth.

While bleaching has been used in dentistry for nearly 200 years, the recent impetus for its use came from the seminal work of Haywood and Heymann in 1989.

Diagnosis of the causes of discolouration, assessment of patients' expectations and full discussion with patients about their available options are all important aspects of bleaching.

Bleaching is now well established as one of the most important appearance-enhancing aspects of modern, evidence-based clinical practice. This book outlines the mechanisms and techniques involved. It also draws attention to some of the pitfalls of dental bleaching and how many of these can be avoided with a sensible, patient-centred, deductive, pragmatic approach.

Bleaching in combination with composite or porcelain bonding can produce results that compare very favourably with much more destructive and expensive traditional crown techniques. Unlike bleaching, many of the alternative more destructive techniques produce negative biological outcomes at considerably greater expense in terms of tooth tissue, time and money.

Bleaching leaves patients with one of their most important assets – good, clean looking, healthy, attractive enamel. Dentists have sought for years to produce natural looking replacements for enamel. Many of the supposedly miraculous porcelain materials produce dismal long-term results. If dentists just had the good sense to leave enamel on the teeth in the first place, there would be many fewer biological and aesthetic problems with teeth in the longer term.

It is prudent to reflect that "less is more" in dentistry. The change away from a destructive mechanical approach to a biological minimally invasive one is to be welcomed. This could be best described as a change from "Meccano to microns" with the gradual realisation that much less damaging dental procedures are worth more to patients than destructive ones. Bleaching in this context, if sensibly applied according to scientifically validated principles, can reasonably be expected to produce good long-term results. This confidence is based on multiple, randomised, double blind, controlled trials.

The book also draws attention to some of the highly publicised but less well proven, if not unsubstantiated, claims made in respect of certain forms and aspects of bleaching.

This book could not have been done without the help of Margaret Buck, who patiently typed all my drafts. My wife Annette provided invaluable (usually constructive) criticism throughout the project.

My thanks are also due to Nairn Wilson for his skilful editorial assistance.

Martin Kelleher

Contents

Chapter 1
Chemistry and Safety of Dental Bleaching

Aim

The aims are to introduce the chemistry of bleaching, to describe how teeth become discoloured and to demonstrate the safety of bleaching techniques.

Outcome

On reading this chapter the practitioner will be more familiar with the chemistry of bleaching discoloured teeth and be reassured as to the safety of dental bleaching.

Introduction

Bleaching is a chemical process involving the oxidation of organic material which is broken down to produce less complex molecules. Most of these smaller molecules are lighter in colour than the original larger molecules. Figs 1-1 and 1-2 show teeth before and after bleaching.

Chemistry

The oxidation/reduction reaction which takes place with bleaching is known as a *redox reaction*. In a redox reaction hydrogen peroxide – the oxidising agent

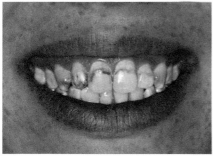

Fig 1-1 Before bleaching.

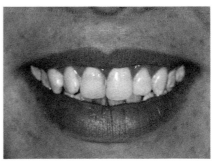

Fig 1-2 After bleaching.

– releases free radicals with unpaired electrons, thereby becoming reduced. The discoloured molecules within the teeth accept the unpaired electrons and become oxidised, with a reduction in the discolouration.

Hydrogen peroxide is an oxidising agent which produces free radicals $HO_2 \cdot$ and $O \cdot$ which are very reactive. The perhydroxyl ion $HO_2 \cdot$ is the stronger and more reactive of the two free radicals. For $HO_2 \cdot$ to be made readily available the bleaching material needs to be alkaline. The optimal pH for $HO_2 \cdot$ release is around pH 10.

Chemistry of Hydrogen Peroxide

The empirical formula for hydrogen peroxide is H_2O_2. The structural formula is HO–OH. The molecular weight of hydrogen peroxide is 34.0.

The empirical formula for carbamide peroxide is $CO(NH_2)_2H_2O_2$. The structural formula is

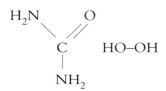

The molecular weight of carbamide peroxide is 94.1.

How Hydrogen Peroxide Works

The whitening effect is caused by the degradation of high molecular weight complex organic molecules that reflect a specific wavelength of light responsible for the colour of the stain. The degradation products have relatively low molecular weights and, as such, are relatively simple and with less colour reflectance. Bleaching results in a reduction or elimination of the discolouration. Both enamel and dentine change colour as a result of the passage of the peroxide through the tooth.

During dental bleaching hydrogen peroxide, which has a low molecular weight, readily penetrates through the interprismatic substance of the enamel to enter dentine and pulp. Because the free radicals have unpaired electrons they readily react with, and attack, most organic molecules. In the process, they generate other radicals. These radicals react with unsaturated bonds, resulting in the disruption of the electron configuration of those molecules. Hydrogen peroxide is capable of undergoing numerous reactions, including molecular additions, substitutions, oxidations and reductions. It is a strong oxidant and can form free radicals by homolytic cleavage.

The various chemical reactions produce a change in the absorption energy of large discoloured molecules within the enamel and dentine. The large molecules are broken down into smaller molecules, with the loss of the unsightly discolouration.

Complex molecules, in particular those forming metallic compounds, look dark whereas simpler molecules look lighter. By breaking down the larger molecules into smaller ones, most are dissipated. Those remaining tend not to have a darkening effect. The result of these various changes is a lighter-looking tooth. In the process of bleaching, highly pigmented carbon ring compounds within the tooth can be broken down and turned into relatively simple chain molecules. Many of these chains have consecutive conjugated double bonds which are further broken into single bonds. These are hydrophilic colourless or lightly pigmented structures.

Theoretically, if bleaching is carried on indefinitely, damage could occur to the enamel matrix. This, however, is largely a theoretical concept. Optimal bleaching involves lightening the teeth to an aesthetically pleasing shade, usually agreed with the patient, while preserving the hardness and strength of the enamel.

How Teeth Become Discoloured

The interprismatic substance between enamel prisms acts like a wick, drawing up ions and small molecules from the oral fluids. Complex molecules – pigments and dyes – stain the interprismatic substance. A pigment is a coloured substance composed of a colour-bearing group (a chromophore) and other molecules. Pigments may, or may not, attach to the organic material in the interprismatic spaces (Fig 1-3).

A dye is a pigment with reactive (hydroxyl or amine) groups which can attach to organic matter (Fig 1-4). Common dyes come from coffee, tea, curry, tomato sauces and red wine. Melanoidins are formed from the break-down products of cooked vegetable oils. Metal compounds can interact with dyes to form larger compounds, which produce different colours of

- A pigment is a coloured substance composed of a colour-bearing group (chromophore) and other molecules

- These may or may not attach to organic material in interprismatic spaces

Fig 1-3 Definition of a pigment.

- A dye is a pigment with reactive groups which can attach itself to the organic matter via -OH or -NH groups, i.e. acidic or basic dyes

- Metal compounds can form with the dye

Fig 1-4 Definition of a dye.

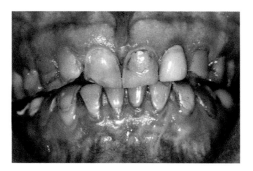

Fig 1-5 Gradual assembly of complex stains within the teeth. Note the contrast with the old crown at the upper left lateral incisor, which previously matched the teeth.

stain. Metal compounds containing iron and copper are often involved (see Figs 1-5 to 1-7).

An increase in the size of a dye increases the affinity of the dye for the organic matter in the interprismatic space. Hydrogen peroxide breaks up large molecular stains into smaller molecules, most of which are expelled through the surface of the tooth. The perhydroxyl ions may attach to molecular stain as well as the protein matrix.

Bleaching produces oxidation which involves the breakdown of ring structures and consecutive, conjugated double bonds in complex molecules. This results in loss of colour caused by unwanted dark molecules in the non-cellular matrix. Hydrogen peroxide works by converting these large molecules into alcohols, ketones and terminal carboxylic acids. As these are smaller molecules which may be expelled from the tooth, the clinical effect is that the tooth is lightened (see Figs 1-8 and 1-9).

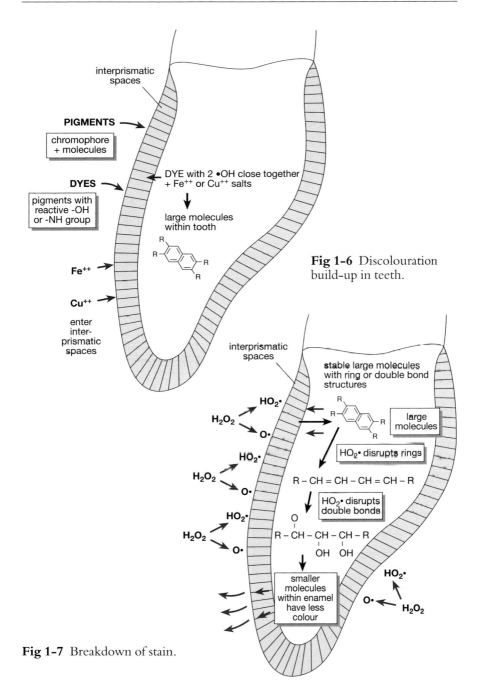

interprismatic
spaces

PIGMENTS
chromophore
+ molecules

DYES
pigments with
reactive -OH
or -NH group

DYE with 2 •OH close together
+ Fe^{++} or Cu^{++} salts

large molecules
within tooth

Fe^{++}

Cu^{++}

enter
inter-
prismatic
spaces

Fig 1-6 Discolouration
build-up in teeth.

interprismatic
spaces

stable large molecules
with ring or double bond
structures

large
molecules

HO$_2$•

H$_2$O$_2$

O•

HO$_2$• disrupts rings

HO$_2$•

H$_2$O$_2$

O•

$R - CH = CH - CH = CH - R$

HO$_2$• disrupts
double bonds

HO$_2$•

H$_2$O$_2$

O•

$R - CH - CH - CH - R$
OH   OH

smaller
molecules
within enamel
have less
colour

HO$_2$•

O•   H$_2$O$_2$

Fig 1-7 Breakdown of stain.

5

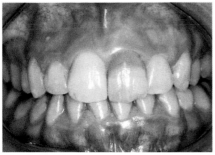 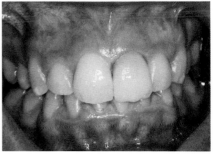

Fig 1-8 Discoloured upper left central incisor before bleaching.

Fig 1-9 Upper left central incisor after bleaching.

Safety of Carbamide Peroxide

Carbamide peroxide is formed from hydrogen peroxide and urea. About one-third of carbamide peroxide is released as hydrogen peroxide. A 10% solution of carbamide peroxide releases about 3.5% hydrogen peroxide (H_2O_2). A 15% solution of carbamide peroxide releases about 5% hydrogen peroxide. Urea is a normal bodily constituent. The urea component of carbamide peroxide used in dental bleaching is of no biological consequence. Hydrogen peroxide is found in all body cells as an endogenous metabolite. The human liver, the principal site of metabolism, produces up to 270 mg of H_2O_2 per hour.

Hydrogen peroxide is rapidly decomposed by enzymes, in particular catalase and various peroxidases. Saliva contains catalase and peroxidases which rapidly break down any hydrogen peroxide released in the mouth during bleaching. These protective mechanisms ensure that the intraoral release of hydrogen peroxide from carbamide peroxide used in dental bleaching has no adverse effects.

All body cells contain enzymes which protect against hydrogen peroxide. The highest levels are found in the liver, duodenum, spleen, blood, mucous membranes and the kidneys. Most of the catalase is found in the red blood cells, which can degrade gram quantities of hydrogen peroxide within a few minutes. The overall decomposition reaction of hydrogen peroxide in the presence of catalase is

$$H_2O_2 + H_2O_2 \rightarrow 2H_2O + O_2 \text{ (water and oxygen)}$$

In the presence of peroxidases the reaction is

$$H_2O_2 + 2RH \rightarrow 2H_2O + R\text{-}R$$

Hydrogen peroxide is broken down into oxygen and water by enzymes such as catalase, peroxidases and selenium-dependent glutathione peroxidases. If any bleaching gel is present in the mouth then the catalase and peroxidase enzymes in saliva will rapidly inactivate it.

Dermal toxicity is low. There is no evidence in the available literature that hydrogen peroxide is a skin sensitiser in humans. Very occasional positive patch tests have been reported.

Biological membranes are highly permeable to hydrogen peroxide. Hydrogen peroxide is readily taken up by the cells of the oral mucosal surfaces, but at the same time it is quickly metabolised. There is uncertainty as to the extent to which hydrogen peroxide enters the bloodstream, given the variable amounts of existing endogenous hydrogen peroxide. In any event, hydrogen peroxide is, as indicated above, rapidly metabolised by red blood cells.

The risk posed by the use of carbamide peroxide for dental bleaching is very small, but there is nothing to which human beings are exposed that is entirely free of risk. The concentration or the dose is the critical issue in any consideration of toxicity. According to toxicologists, "the dose makes the poison". Provided that the concentration of hydrogen peroxide is low and the dose is small, any risk of adverse reaction is very limited.

The toxicology of hydrogen peroxide was reviewed by the International Association for Research on Cancer (IARC) in 1985, by the European Centre for Ecotoxicology and Toxicology of Chemicals (ECETOC) in 1993 and by Li in 2003. These reviews concluded that there are no reasons for concern about the use of hydrogen peroxide in the concentrations employed in dentist-prescribed at-home bleaching.

Sensitivity
Temporary dentine hypersensitivity is a well-known adverse effect of bleaching. Approximately 70% of patients experience some sensitivity during nightguard vital bleaching with 10% carbamide peroxide. This sensitivity is very mild and transitory, persisting for up to 24 hours following the completion of bleaching. Increased sensitivity is mainly associated with

7

the use of heat and high concentrations of hydrogen peroxide in attempts to accelerate the bleaching process.

Soft Tissues

The American Dental Association Guidelines for the acceptance of peroxide products were published in 1994 (see www.ada.org/ada/seal/standards/guidehome_bleach.pdf). These guidelines require an evaluation of the effects of bleaching on the soft tissues of the mouth, including the tongue, lips, palate and gingivae.

To date, none of the published studies on the use of 10% carbamide peroxide have reported any adverse effects on soft tissues. When mild transient damage to gingival tissues has occurred, it appears to have been related to trauma caused by a poorly fitting tray.

In nightguard vital bleaching, during which the carbamide peroxide is effectively contained within a customised tray, the risk of adverse effects on soft tissues is very limited.

Tooth Resorption

There are no reports of 10% carbamide peroxide (3.5% hydrogen peroxide) causing resorption, let alone other damage to enamel or dentine, when used for internal or inside/outside bleaching.

Resorption frequently occurs as a result of trauma to teeth. The severity is related to the type of injury sustained, the force involved and whether the tooth was dislodged, intruded or laterally luxated. Severe damage or excessive drying of the periodontal ligament, damage to cementum, contamination of the root, and failure to root fill or splint appropriately, all increase the risks of resorption of a traumatised tooth.

Cervical resorption is very occasionally seen in bleached, root-filled teeth, but only when a high concentration of hydrogen peroxide (30–38%) is applied in conjunction with heat to the already damaged tooth surfaces.

Pulpal Considerations

Hydrogen peroxide penetrates readily and quickly to the dental pulp. The higher the concentration the more rapidly it appears in the pulp. Following exposure to hydrogen peroxide, histological studies have shown a mild inflammatory response. The mild inflammation appears to be limited to the superficial layers of the pulp immediately subjacent to the dentopulpal junction. These observations are consistent with the mild discomfort reported by patients as early as 15 minutes following exposure to hydrogen peroxide for the purpose of bleaching.

Despite the uptake of hydrogen peroxide, the pulp suffers no irreversible damage as a consequence of bleaching. Even following the use of 40% hydrogen peroxide in chair-side bleaching, the pulpal damage is reversible. There are no reports of teeth dying, even with very prolonged (6–9 months) use of 10% carbamide peroxide.

Effects on Hardness of Teeth

There are numerous laboratory studies (Haywood et al., 1990; McCracken and Haywood, 1996; Teixeria et al., 2004) which show that peroxide-containing tooth-whitening products do not affect the microstructure of enamel. The abrasion resistance of enamel is not lowered by bleaching, nor is the microhardness or mineral content altered.

Likewise, the microhardness of dental restorations is not affected. The critical pH for teeth is 5.5; below this pH teeth tend to erode. As the vast majority of carbamide peroxide products have a pH of 6.5–7 then even if a high concentration of hydrogen peroxide is used, there is no reduction in the hardness of enamel or dentine, let alone dissolution of tooth structure.

Amalgam Restorations

Laboratory studies, employing exaggerated conditions, have demonstrated release of very small amounts of mercury from dental amalgam restorations. However, the levels of release are well within the limits of mercury exposure established by the World Health Organization (WHO) and do not pose a risk to patients. Notwithstanding these findings, it is prudent to replace any amalgam restorations in anterior teeth with temporary tooth-coloured restorations prior to bleaching (Figs 1-10 and 1-11). This will avoid the very limited risk of producing a green discolouration caused by the corrosion of copper in amalgam restorations.

Tooth-coloured Restorative Materials

Tooth-coloured restorative materials do not bleach. Consequently, any tooth-coloured restorations may appear darker following bleaching. It is important for a dentist to discuss this matter with patients before they agree to bleach. Patients are frequently unaware of which of their teeth have restorations.

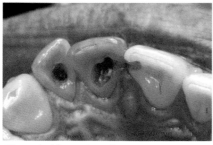

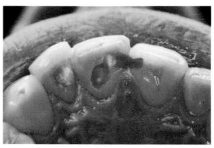

Fig 1-10 Amalgam restorations removed prior to bleaching.

Fig 1-11 Temporary restorations covering root fillings.

Most of the over-the-counter bleaching products do not warn of the possibility of colour mismatch between existing restorations and remaining tooth tissue (see Chapter 6). Patients who have used such products may present requesting the replacement of dark, unaesthetic restorations. There are "bleached" shades of composite available which may be necessary if teeth are very white.

Adhesive Bonds and Rebound

Bond strengths between enamel and resin-based fillings are reduced for the first 24 hours after bleaching. Thereafter, there is no difference in the bond strengths of composite resin to bleached or non-bleached enamel.

Rebound is a term used in bleaching to describe changes in the colour of teeth after bleaching. These effects are linked to the loss of oxygen from teeth and any associated rehydration if the teeth have been isolated under rubber dam. Rebound, while largely completed in the first 24 hours after bleaching, may take up to seven days to complete. Therefore it is prudent to delay post-bleaching restorative procedures.

Bonding of teeth should be delayed to ensure good colour matching and optimal bond strength. This is especially important when placing indirect restorations such as porcelain veneers as any residual oxygen within the teeth could produce oxygen inhibition of the composite luting cement. When planning such restorations, as a precautionary measure it is sensible to confiscate the bleaching tray from the patient ahead of the preparation stage. In this way the patient will not be able to bleach their teeth between preparation and fitting of definitive restorations.

The patient should also be advised not to use any sort of over-the-counter bleaching product during this time, as this will adversely affect bond strengths and possibly the colour match.

Chair-side Bleaching

Chair-side bleaching is done in the dental chair using relatively high concentrations of hydrogen peroxide (15–38%). Bearing in mind that 25% hydrogen peroxide is equivalent to 75% carbamide peroxide and 38% hydrogen peroxide is equivalent to 114% carbamide peroxide, the chair-side bleaching strength is up to 11 times the concentration of the 10% carbamide peroxide material normally used for nightguard vital bleaching.

It is important to recognise that chair-side bleaching can cause soft tissue damage. To avoid such damage, strenuous efforts are required to protect all soft tissues of the patient: the use of rubber dam is essential. Damage appears as a white burn of the epithelium and such burns are painful. This sloughs off leaving a red, painful ulcerated area.

In the event of an adverse soft tissue reaction, the area should be washed thoroughly and the patient reassured. The painful area normally takes a week to ten days to heal. Scarring is not usually a problem, as the ulceration is superficial. Eye protection is essential for patients and all members of the dental team throughout chair-side bleaching.

Unfounded Fears

Fears that the use of carbamide peroxide poses a risk of malignant change in oral soft tissues are unfounded. The concentrations of carbamide peroxide used in bleaching teeth do not carry any risk of mutagenesis in humans.

At-risk Groups

The only individuals known to be at any risk from bleaching with hydrogen peroxide are patients with very rare conditions such as acatalasaemia or glucose-6-phosphate dehydrogenase (G6PD) deficiency. This makes them more susceptible to peroxide activity.

Acatalasaemia is a rare (0.2%) condition. It is an inherited disease in which there is a deficiency of catalase. G6PD is a disorder of erythrocytes in which the metabolic problems of the affected cells result in inadequate

11

detoxification of hydrogen peroxide. The frequency of G6PD deficiency in Europe is about 0.1%.

Efficacy and Effectiveness

ADA guidelines for bleaching are very strict. They require manufacturers to show both the safety-in-use of products and their efficacy. The data required include:

- Findings from two randomised prospective double-blind clinical trials, involving the comparison of the test material with a non-active control material.
- The assessment of the effects of treatment over a period of two to six weeks.
- The measurement of tooth colour at the start and end of treatment using two different systems of colour measurement.
- Three- and six-month colour duration measurements to assess whether the colour improvement is maintained. It also requires that 85% of any colour change is maintained at three months and 75% of colour change is maintained at six months.

A current list of approved products is available from the ADA website: www.ada.org/ada/seal/company_professional.asp.

Mouth Rinses

Over-the-counter mouth rinses such as Bocasan (Oral B, Gillette Group) and Peroxyl (Colgate Palmolive) are freely available. Bocasan releases about 7% hydrogen peroxide and Peroxyl contains 1.5% hydrogen peroxide. The concentrations of hydrogen peroxide in mouth rinses do not bleach teeth. They may, however, have some minor, short-term beneficial effect on oral hygiene and possibly the management of certain extrinsic stains.

References

American Dental Association Council on Dental Therapeutics. Guidelines for the acceptance of peroxide-containing oral hygiene products. J Am Dent Assoc 1994;125:1140-1142.

European Centre for Ecotoxicology and Toxicology of Chemicals. Joint Assessment of Commodity Chemicals No. 22: Hydrogen Peroxide (CAS No. 7722-84-1). ECETOC, Brussels 1993.

Haywood VB, Leech T, Heymann HO et al. Nightguard vital bleaching: effects on enamel surface texture and diffusion. In: Operative dentistry. Quintessence Int. 1990;801-804.

International Association for Research on Cancer. Hydrogen peroxide: evaluation of the carcinogenic risk of chemicals to humans. IARC 1985;36:285–314.

Li Y. The safety of peroxide-containing at-home tooth whiteners. Compend Contin Educ Dent 2003;24:384–389.

McCracken MS, Haywood VB. Demineralization effects of 10 percent carbamide peroxide. J Dent 1996;24:395-398.

Teixeira EC, Ritrer AV, Thompson JY et al. Effect of tray-based and trayless tooth whitening systems on microhardness of enamel surface and subsurface. J Am Dent Assoc 2004;17:433-436.

Further Reading

Cooper JS, Bokmeyer TJ, Bowles WH. Penetration of the pulp chamber by carbamide peroxide bleaching agents. J Endod 1992;18:315–317.

Feinman RA, Madray G, Yarborough D. Chemical, optical and physiologic mechanisms of bleaching products: a review. Pract Periodontics Aesthet Dent 1991;3:32–36.

Frysh H. Chemistry of bleaching. In: Goldstein RE, Garber DA (eds) Complete Dental Bleaching. Quintessence Books, 1995;25.

Haywood VB. History, safety and effectiveness of current bleaching techniques and applications of the nightguard vital bleaching technique. Quintessence Int 1992;23:471–488.

Heithersay GS, Dahlstrom SW, Marin PD. Incidence of invasive cervical resorption in bleached root-filled teeth. Aust Dent J 1994;39:82–87.

Heymann HO. Nonrestorative treatment of discolored teeth; reports from an International Symposium. Univ of Chapel Hill, North Carolina. J Am Dent Assoc 1997;128(suppl):1S–64S.

Kelleher MG, Roe FJ. The safety-in-use of 10% carbamide peroxide (Opalescence) for bleaching teeth under the supervision of a dentist. Br Dent J 1999;187:190–194.

Schulte JR, Morrissette DB, Gasior EJ et al. The effects of bleaching application time on the dental pulp. J Am Dent Assoc 1994;125:1330–1335.

Sterrett J, Price RB, Bankey T. Effects of home bleaching on the tissues of the oral cavity. J Can Dent Assoc 1995;61:412–417:420.

Chapter 2
Nightguard Vital Bleaching

Aim

The aim of this chapter is to consider the indications for nightguard vital bleaching and to outline the technique. Tray design and issues pertaining to existing restorations are covered.

Outcome

On reading this chapter the practitioner will be familiar with the pre-bleaching assessment of patients, the protocol for nightguard vital bleaching, and tray design.

Introduction

Nightguard vital bleaching has revolutionised aesthetic dentistry in that it produces a safe, effective and scientifically proven method of improving the appearance of discoloured teeth.

Development

The most popular, predictable and well-researched method of bleaching teeth is *nightguard vital bleaching*. This technique was developed by Haywood and Heymann in 1989. With this method, 10% carbamide peroxide is placed in a customised tray which is worn by the patient while asleep, hence the expression nightguard vital bleaching.

Haywood and Heymann were largely responsible for the clinical development and the scientific evaluation of nightguard vital bleaching. They based the development on earlier work by Klusmier, Wagner, Austin and Munro. Klusmier was an orthodontist, Wagner a paedodontist, Austin a general dentist and Munro a periodontist. Working independently, these individuals noted lightening of teeth as a side-effect of using carbamide peroxide in the management of gingival tissue conditions. It was Haywood, however, who made bleaching more widely available, following rigorous scientific evaluation.

The most acceptable evidence for good clinical practice is based on the results of prospective, randomised, double-blind, controlled clinical trials. Such trials are relatively rare in dentistry but a number of such trials have confirmed the safety and efficacy of nightguard vital bleaching. Colour changes have been reported to be maintained over periods of up to four years. Figs 2-1 and 2-2 show examples of teeth before and after bleaching.

Patient Management

All dental procedures have advantages and disadvantages. Assessment of patient expectations of bleaching is extremely important and should be done at the earliest opportunity. With nightguard vital bleaching the main clinical issue is compliance in wearing the tray with the bleaching gel in it for the required periods of time.

If patients indicate an interest in bleaching, it is good practice to have information packs available. These packs can be e-mailed or posted to patients prior to their consultation in order to give them basic information on bleaching and time to reflect on the advantages and disadvantages ahead of the consultation appointment.

There is no reason to avoid the use of occlusal coverage trays in patients with a history of temperomandibular joint dysfunction (TMD). It is prudent, however, to warn patients with a history of TMD that they may experience some mild discomfort. There are no reports of patients undergoing nightguard vital bleaching complaining of TMD during the bleaching process. In fact, some TMD patients may experience some relief of their symptoms, given that the soft bleaching tray may double as a soft TMD guard.

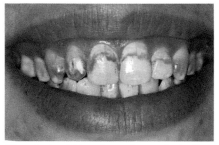

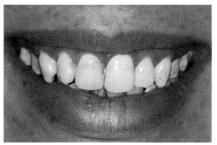

Fig 2-1 Discoloured teeth before bleaching.

Fig 2-2 Teeth after bleaching.

Pre-examination Questionnaire

A patient pre-examination questionnaire may be a useful adjunct prior to the consultation. This should include questions such as:

- What do you wish to achieve?
- Have you tried any other treatment for your teeth? If so, how did you find the results?
- What do you think has caused the problem?
- What would you consider a satisfactory solution?
  (Please note, if somebody answers "very white" be careful, as their expectations may be too high. "Somewhat lighter teeth" is a much more realistic treatment objective.)
- How long do you think treatment may take to achieve the desired result?

Protocol

The protocol for nightguard vital bleaching is based on that developed by Haywood and Heymann and is as follows:

- A history is taken, a detailed clinical examination carried out and a differential diagnosis is made in respect of the cause of the discolouration.
- Restorations in the target and adjacent teeth are recorded. Veneers or crowns are charted as these, together with other existing restorations, will not change colour with bleaching.
- A note is made as to whether the periodontal tissues are thick or thin (Fig 2-3).
- A three-in-one syringe is used to blow air around the teeth to be bleached and any sensitivity recorded. Patients should be warned that if any teeth are sensitive at the time of initial examination then these teeth are likely to get much more sensitive with bleaching (Fig 2-4). Patients presenting

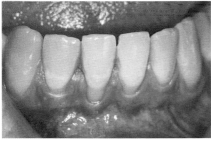

Fig 2-3 Thin periodontal tissues. Note the dehiscence at the lower right central incisor.

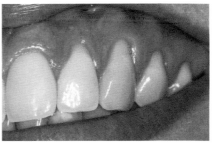

Fig 2-4 Recession at the upper left lateral incisor and canine. These teeth are likely to be sensitive when bleaching.

with sensitivity may need to bleach for two hours only at a time, rather than for the typical overnight period.

- Tooth surface loss caused by, in particular, erosion is noted as the affected teeth may be sensitive and become more sensitive with bleaching (Fig 2-5). Tooth wear due to attrition is rarely a problem when bleaching.

- The shade of the teeth is agreed with the patient by reference to a value-oriented (from light to dark) shade guide. This shade is recorded in the notes and a written record given to the patient.

- The patient's expectations, whether they are realistic or not, need to be assessed. If a patient whose teeth are already very white insists that they are too dark, it is probably unwise to proceed with bleaching. A diagnosis of possible dysmorphophobia (distortion of body image) should be considered.

- The option of bleaching just one arch rather than both arches should be discussed with the patient.

- Any abnormalities of enamel and dentine, the extent and sufficiency of any restorations and the presence or absence of any periodontal conditions are noted (see Fig 2-6).

- Radiographs, if appropriate and indicated, are taken and a note made of any relevant findings, including periapical status, sclerosis, atypical pulp morphology or size (see Fig 2-7).

- A check on whether the patient retches can be made by running a finger along the expected extension of the bleaching tray. If patients retch, or are unable to tolerate having an appliance in their mouth for prolonged periods while awake or asleep, then nightguard vital bleaching is unlikely to be successful. Frequently, patients who retch have a history of having had an invasive procedure such as tonsillectomy or extraction of teeth

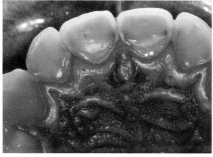

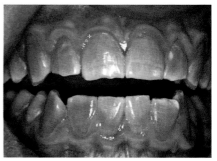

Fig 2-5 Erosion of the palatal aspects of the upper incisors. These teeth are likely to be sensitive when bleaching.

Fig 2-6 A case of dentinogenesis imperfecta.

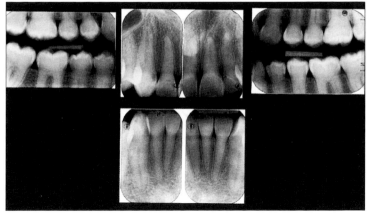

Fig 2-7 Radiographs reveal the absence of pulp chambers and canals.

under general anaesthesia. Patients who have experienced a difficult general anaesthetic frequently show great reluctance to have an appliance in their mouth. It is prudent to discuss such details as part of the patient's history, prior to incurring the costs of making bleaching trays. Retching when an impression is being taken may be a warning of future difficulties with compliance.

- A photograph is taken of the teeth to be bleached and the opposing teeth, with a shade guide tab being held adjacent to the teeth as a reference (Fig 2-8).

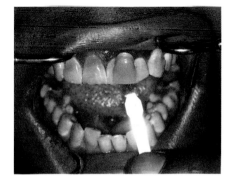

Fig 2-8 The shade tab is held beside the teeth when the preoperative photograph is taken. This acts as a reference to monitor changes during bleaching.

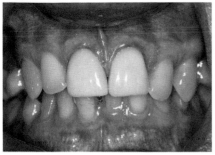

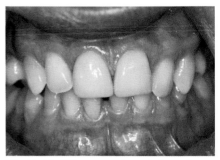

Fig 2-9 Dark teeth before bleaching with lighter crowns present on the upper central incisors.

Fig 2-10 The natural teeth have been bleached to match the crowns. The crowns have not changed colour.

- The alternatives to bleaching are discussed. Attention is drawn to the fact that restorations will not change colour. This is a very important aspect of consent for bleaching. If this is not done before bleaching is started patients may think that their restorations are getting darker or otherwise damaged as their natural teeth are becoming lighter.
- Patients may blame the dentist for changing the colour of their restorations and expect these to be replaced free of charge. The clinical and laboratory costs of replacing restorations can easily exceed the cost of bleaching. The apportionment of the costs of such treatment can be the subject of dispute.
- If veneers, crowns, bridges or implant-retained crowns are lighter, the patient should be advised that bleaching can lighten the natural teeth to match the restorations (Figs 2-9 and 2-10).

If the natural teeth are lighter than adjacent crowns/veneers then bleaching will make things look worse. Patients with existing restorations need to be warned to control the rate of bleaching and not to overbleach the natural teeth. It is prudent to limit the amount of bleaching gel given to such patients and to review them at one-week intervals.

Patients need to be told that if the natural teeth start to go lighter than the restorations, they must stop bleaching immediately and return to the surgery for reassessment (Figs 2-11 and 2-12).

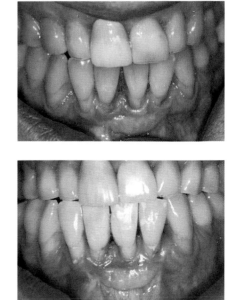

Fig 2-11 Existing crown on the upper right central incisor with discoloured adjacent and opposing teeth.

Fig 2-12 Teeth adjacent to and opposing the crowned upper right central incisor have been bleached. The colour of the crown has not changed. Direct composite bonding has been used to reduce the gaps between the lower teeth. Note that the existing free gingival graft has not been affected.

Clinical Procedures

- An alginate impression of the teeth is taken. It is advisable to use a finger to wipe some alginate around all the occlusal and labial aspects of the teeth prior to insertion of the loaded tray. This minimises the formation of air bubbles and helps produce an accurate cast. This, in turn, will allow a well-fitting tray to be constructed. Any air bubbles in the impression appear as positives on the cast. The tray will have corresponding voids over non-target areas where the bleaching gel will accumulate in an unplanned way.
- The teeth to be bleached are identified on the laboratory instruction card, together with an indication of the outline and extension of the tray (see Fig 2-13 for an example of teeth damaged by tetracycline). The teeth to be bleached are blocked out with plaster or resin (see the section on tray design below). This is usually done for each tooth on the cast from one first molar to the other first molar.

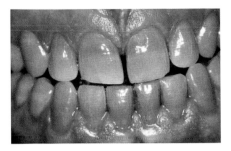

Fig 2-13 Teeth discoloured by tetracycline prior to impressions.

- The thickness of the material to be used in the construction of the tray is specified. The tray material should be strong in thin section. A 1 mm clear preheated blank is usually suitable. If the patient is a bruxist, a thicker material (2 mm) is indicated. The material should be easily adapted and capable of being finished to a smooth edge to prevent trauma to the gingival tissues and tongue. It should be non-allergenic, stable, and easy to clean. Softray (Ultradent Products Inc.) which is 0.8 mm thick is a suitable material for most cases.

Tray Design

The purpose of the tray is to hold the bleaching gel in contact with the teeth to be bleached. Different designs of tray are indicated depending on the viscosity of the bleaching gel. Poorly designed or badly made trays will not produce the desired outcome.

Trays with Reservoirs

Trays used for nightguard vital bleaching normally have reservoirs. The purpose of the reservoirs is to retain the bleaching gel in the desired areas. If more gel is required over a particularly dark part of a tooth, this area can be preferentially blocked out (see Figs 2-14 to 2-16). An alternative approach, using composite applied directly to the teeth prior to taking the impressions, is outlined in Chapter 4.

The need for a reservoir is largely dependent on the viscosity of the bleaching material. Carboxypolymethylcellulose (carbopol) is a thickening agent which is added to carbamide peroxide. The increased viscosity limits movement of the gel. It is important to be able to seat the tray and still keep the bleaching gel in the correct position. It is impossible to compress a gel; it can only be displaced.

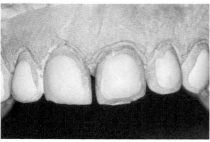

Fig 2-14 Cast blocked out with plaster.

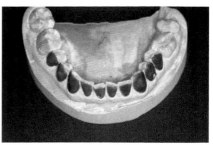

Fig 2-15 Occlusal view of cast blocked out with resin.

Fig 2-16 Tray extending from the lower right first permanent molar to the lower left first permanent molar on the blocked-out cast.

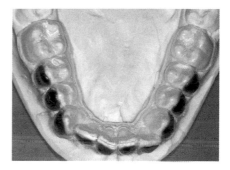

It is important to design the tray so as to avoid gel coming into unnecessary contact with soft tissues. The reservoirs allow perhydroxyl ions released from the carbamide peroxide to pass preferentially through the darkest discoloured areas of the teeth.

The bleaching effect cannot be limited to the reservoir areas. However, reservoirs help to ensure that most of the bleaching gel is held over the target areas.

The presence of reservoirs helps the loaded tray to seat fully on the teeth. If the tray does not seat properly, it will usually be short at the gingival margins. This may result in a failure to bleach the necks of teeth. If the necks of the teeth are not covered by the tray then salivary peroxidases and catalase can react with the unprotected gel and rapidly inactivate the hydrogen peroxide.

23

Some commentators have suggested that reservoirs are unnecessary and that trays without reservoirs are more economical. Trays with reservoirs can indeed be bulkier and need more bleaching material. The counter-argument is that if there is an inadequate amount of bleaching gel in the target areas then trays without reservoirs are a false economy. Keeping saliva away from the gel helps keep it active for longer. Reservoirs hold the bleaching gel in the tray for several hours and this allows the gel to continue releasing perhydroxyl ions to sustain the bleaching process.

If there is a veneer on the labial aspect of the tooth, the reservoir should be on the palatal aspect of the tray, as the gel will not penetrate the veneering material. The peroxide will, however, penetrate through the palatal enamel, palatal dentine and dental pulp to reach, albeit slowly, the dentine of the labial aspect of the tooth. In this way veneered teeth can be lightened.

The viscous nature of the bleaching gel has added advantages. If the tray is unretentive on its own it can become retentive once the gel is placed in it. Viscous 10% carbamide peroxide materials such as Opalescence (Ultradent Products Inc.) are designed for use with a reservoir.

The block-out material used to create the reservoirs is generally placed on the buccal aspects of the teeth on the cast. Blocking out should stop about 1 mm short of the incisal tip (Fig 2-17). The incisal tip is mainly enamel and this area bleaches readily without the need for a reservoir.

The reservoirs can be of different sizes, depending on the specific circumstances. The more bulbous or darker the tooth the greater is the need for a reservoir. If the necks of teeth are to be bleached, the reservoirs should extend over the gingival margin, but in such a way that the tray does not pinch the soft tissues but is still capable of holding the gel in the cervical regions. In such cases it is prudent to check that the patient does not have thin, friable periodontal tissues that may be traumatised by the extended tray (see Figs 2-3 and 2-4).

Contraindications for this method of bleaching are very limited width of thin attached gingiva and marked preoperative cervical sensitivity. These conditions also restrict alternative treatments, limiting the opportunity to satisfy certain patients' demands for bleaching of their teeth.

Scalloped Trays
Scalloped trays (Figs 2-17 and 2-18) follow the gingival margins. When the tray material has been adapted to the model a permanent ink pen can be used

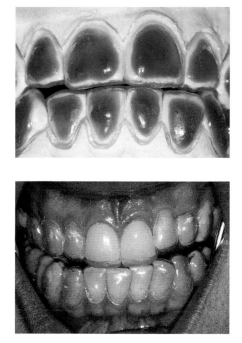

Fig 2-17 Scalloped trays with reservoirs on the labial aspects. The material used for blocking out stops short of the incisal tips.

Fig 2-18 Scalloped trays in position. The porcelain veneers on the upper central incisors are not covered by the tray.

to draw the outline of the underlying gingival margins on the labial aspect of the clear tray material. The tray is then removed from the cast and cut along this outline with a pair of sharp scissors. Scissors have been specifically designed for this purpose (Ultradent Products Inc.) and they can produce a tray with a smooth edge which is well tolerated by the tongue. If the scalloping is positioned short of the gingival margin some gel will extrude over the gingival tissues. This gel will be quickly inactivated by salivary catalase and peroxidases and consequently the necks of the teeth may fail to bleach.

One disadvantage of scalloped trays is that some patients find the margins on the lingual/palatal aspects irritating to the tongue, even when suitably finished.

Straight-line Trays
Straight-line trays have been advocated on the grounds that they are easy to construct and hold an appropriate volume of bleaching material over the cervical margins of the teeth. These trays extend about 2 mm beyond the gingival margins. An advantage of straight-line trays is that they tend not to irritate

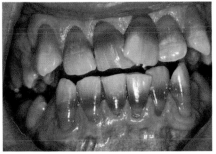

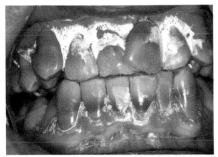

Fig 2-19 Crowded anterior teeth with marked banded tetracycline discolouration.

Fig 2-20 Straight-line trays in position.

the tongue. A disadvantage is that by having bleaching material held over the gingival tissues there may be a mild, transient soft tissue reaction to the gel.

Reservoirs are indicated with this type of tray. They can be placed on the palatal as well as the labial aspects of the teeth, although this can make the tray somewhat bulky (Figs 2-19 and 2-20).

Single-tooth Trays
Single-tooth trays are designed to bleach individual teeth. In such cases, a standard tray is adjusted by trimming it away from the labial aspect of the adjacent teeth. By cutting away the tray, the salivary enzymes inactivate any hydrogen peroxide coming in contact with the adjacent teeth, which will not therefore bleach. This is especially important, for example, when bleaching a single dark tooth (see Figs 2-21 and 2-22 and Chapter 3).

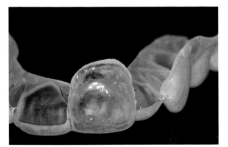

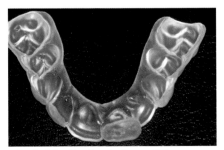

Fig 2-21 Close-up of the labial aspect of a single-tooth tray.

Fig 2-22 Occlusal view of the extension of a single-tooth tray.

Combination Trays

Combination trays are used in situations where, for example, it is planned to bleach the canines and one central incisor only. A combination tray is produced by modifying a standard tray to hold the gel over the target teeth only. Cutting windows makes a tray less retentive and relatively flimsy. It is important to incorporate retention in such trays by extending the tray into normal undercuts in the premolar and molar regions (Fig 2-16).

Technical Procedures

- An alginate impression is taken of the teeth (Fig 2-23) and an accurate plaster cast of the arch to be bleached is produced. The plaster cast should be horseshoe-shaped and have sufficient bulk to ensure adequate strength. The base of the cast is trimmed to be parallel to the occlusal plane.
- Block-out resin is placed over the target teeth and light-cured in position (Fig 2-24).
- Cold-mould seal is applied to the cast to help with the removal of the vacuum formed thermoplastic material.

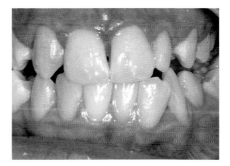

Fig 2-23 The upper right canine is in the position of the upper right lateral incisor and is not symmetric with the upper left lateral incisor. The upper left canine is missing.

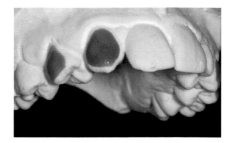

Fig 2-24 Target teeth blocked out with resin on the cast.

27

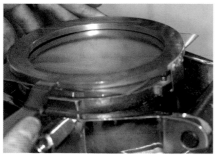

Fig 2-25 The thermoplastic material is heated.

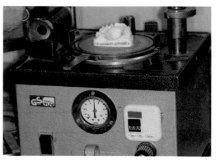

Fig 2-26 The cast on the table of the vacuum-forming machine with the occlusal aspects facing upwards.

- The thermoplastic material is made of ethyl vinyl acetate and comes in various thicknesses. If there is clinical evidence of tooth wear, or parafunctional activity, a relatively thick sheet of material should be used.
- The modified cast is placed on the platform with the occlusal aspect facing the plastic sheet. The thermoplastic material is heated until it goes clear and is then adapted to the cast in a vacuum-forming machine (Figs 2-25 and 2-26).

Following adaptation, the tray material is allowed to cool (Fig 2-27).

- Excess material is removed with sharp scissors and a scalpel. If the necks of the teeth are dark, the material is trimmed back so that it just covers the gingival tissues on the cast. Check for any sharp edges with a finger.

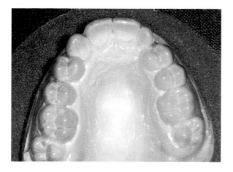

Fig 2-27 Bleaching tray material adapted to the cast.

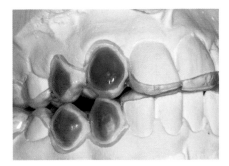

Fig 2-28 The trays have been modified to bleach the right canine and first premolar teeth and to avoid bleaching the upper and lower incisors.

- Finish the tray with burs, a scalpel and appropriate polishing systems. Fig 2-28 shows trays that have been adapted.

Fitting the Tray

- The fit of the tray is checked. There should be no blanching of the soft tissues. This is especially important to check if the gingival tissues are thin and may be damaged by ill-fitting or sharp margins. The patient should be asked to identify any uncomfortable areas with their tongue. These areas should be adjusted as necessary.
- The teeth to be bleached can be marked on the outer surface of the tray with a permanent felt tip pen (Fig 2-29). This helps the patient identify where to place the bleaching gel.
- The accuracy of the photographs obtained at the initial appointment is checked with the patient and then replaced in the notes. The agreed shade

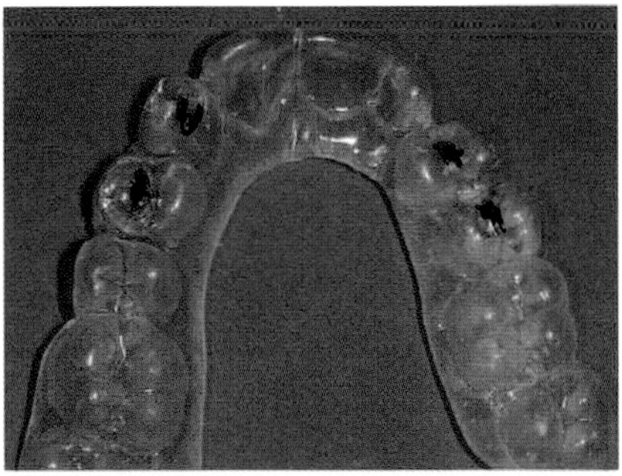

Fig 2-29 The target teeth marked with a permanent felt tip pen on the outside of the tray.

29

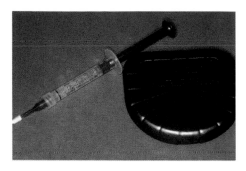

Fig 2-30 Container for the storage of tray.

is confirmed with reference to the value-orientated shade guide (arranged from lightest to darkest) and confirmed in the clinical record. The patient is given a note of the agreed existing shade of the teeth.

- The appropriate amount of 10% carbamide peroxide is given to the patient along with written instructions. Higher concentrations of carbamide peroxide bleaching gel may be prescribed but there is little scientific evidence of real benefits in doing so. Higher concentrations can produce a more rapid response in some patients but there is also sometimes an increased risk of sensitivity.
- The patient is given a protective (orthodontic retainer style) box for safe storage of the bleaching trays when not in use (Fig 2-30).
- A log form should be given to the patient to record the use of the bleaching trays and the amount of material used.
- Patients who experience any sensitivity of their teeth can be advised to use toothpaste containing 5% potassium nitrate (KNO_3). This can be used two weeks prior to bleaching, or it can be placed in the tray and worn for half an hour before each bleaching session. Five per cent potassium nitrate materials are available specifically to reduce sensitivity (Ultra Eeze, Ultradent Products Inc.). This material has the same viscosity as 10% carbamide peroxide.

Evaluation of Colour Change

Photographs should be taken to record changes in colour. All changes should be recorded in the patient's clinical records.

A clinical record checklist for bleaching should include the following information with dates:

- Diagnosis   Y/N
- Radiographs   Y/N
- Photographs   Y/N
- Discussion of options with patient   Y/N
- Discuss option of single-arch bleaching   Y/N
- Consent   Y/N
- Impressions   Y/N
- Mouthguard inserted   Date
- Material used and quantity
- Time of recall

Figs 2-31 and 2-32 show examples of one arch bleaching.

Instructions for Patients for the Use of 10% Carbamide Peroxide

1. Brush your teeth thoroughly in the normal fashion.
2. Remove the tip from the syringe containing the 10% carbamide peroxide gel and extrude a little of the contents into the appropriate parts of the tray towards the deeper and front parts of the mould of each tooth to be bleached.
3. Place gel in the tray on the cheek and the tongue side of the back teeth. About half to three quarters of the syringe will usually be necessary.
4. Seat the tray over the teeth and slowly press down firmly.
5. A finger, a tissue, or a soft toothbrush should be used to remove excess gel that will flow beyond the edge of the tray.
6. Rinse gently – do not swallow. The tray is usually worn overnight while sleeping but as long as it is worn for at least 2 hours, this will be effective.
7. In the morning remove the tray and brush the residual gel from the teeth. Rinse out the tray and brush it to remove the residual gel. Store it in a safe container.

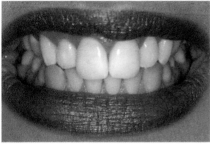 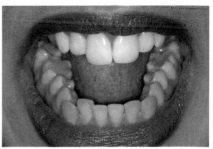

Fig 2-31 Patient with upper arch bleached.

Fig 2-32 Contrast between upper and lower arches.

8. One or both trays can be worn overnight. However, if bleaching both upper and lower teeth it is preferable to bleach one arch at night and the other for at least 2 hours during the day.
9. Do not eat, drink or smoke while wearing the bleaching tray.
10. Carbamide peroxide should not be exposed to heat, sunlight or extreme cold.

Notes
1. It is counterproductive to apply the bleaching gel more than once a day, as this has been shown to increase sensitivity, which in turn tends to delay completion of bleaching.
2. It will probably take about three to four weeks to achieve a satisfactory result. Your dentist will advise you but the general rule is to keep bleaching until the teeth are an acceptable colour.

Sensitivity
About 70% of patients experience significant sensitivity while bleaching. If this happens then bleaching should be stopped for a day or two and recommenced on an every second or every third night basis. Fluoride gel or toothpaste can be used to treat sensitive teeth. This can be placed in the tray and worn at night. Toothpaste with 5% potassium nitrate will probably be more effective at reducing sensitivity than other sensitivity toothpastes. Acidic drinks and fruit should be avoided as these are known to cause sensitivity. Very rarely temporary discomfort of the gums, lips and tongue can occur. These usually reduce dramatically once bleaching stops.

Rebleaching
Rebleaching normally takes one night for each week of the original course. If it took three weeks to bleach initially it will take three days to "top up".

Bleaching dos and don'ts for the dentist

Do ...
- Take a history. Record the shade in the notes.
- Make a diagnosis of what is causing the discolouration.
- Discuss the options.
- Discuss the costs.
- Discuss the estimated treatment time.
- Discuss the time to "top up".
- Check for secondary "flecking" (white spots) in fluorosis.

put in notes

- Check if there is retching.
- Block out casts as appropriate.
- Control the amount of bleach issued.
- Have advice sheets on alternative treatments, e.g. veneers.
- Check for the presence of composites.
- Check on the radiographs for composites.
- Warn that composites will not bleach and will have to be replaced.
- Check for the presence of veneers, crowns, bridges.
- Warn that these will not bleach and may need to be redone when the natural teeth change colour.
- Keep **high-concentration hydrogen peroxide** products separate from standard carbamide peroxide products.

put in notes

Don't ...
- Promise the earth.
- Encourage patients to use stronger concentrations or change the gel more than once a day.
- Believe unsubstantiated manufacturers' claims.
- Use non-CE-marked products.
- Use non-ADA-approved bleaching products.
- Believe all products are the same.
- Delegate the distribution of extra bleaching material to staff without checking.

Reference

Haywood VB, Heymann HO. Nightguard vital bleaching. Quintessence Int 1989;20:173–176.

Further Reading

Haywood VB, Leonard RH, Neilson CF, Brunson WD. Effectiveness, side effects and long-term status of nightguard vital bleaching. J Am Dent Assoc 1994;125:1219–1226.

Leonard RH Jr, Bentley C, Eagle JC, Garland GE, Knight MC, Phillips C. Nightguard vital bleaching: a long term study on efficacy, shade retention, side effects, and patient perceptions. J Esthet Restor Dent 2001;13:357–369.

Leonard RH, Haywood VB, Caplan DJ, Tart ND. Nightguard vital bleaching of tetracycline-stained teeth: 90 months post treatment. J Esthet Restor Dent 2003;15:142–152.

Matis BA, Hamdan YS, Cochran MA, Eckert GJ. A clinical evaluation of a bleaching agent used with and without reservoirs. Oper Dent 2002;27:5–11.

Matis BA, Wang Y, Jiang T, Eckert GJ. Extended at-home bleaching of tetracycline-stained teeth with different combinations of carbamide peroxide. Quintessence Int 2002;33:645–655.

Ritter AV, Leonard RH, St George AJ et al. Safety and stability of nightguard vital bleaching 9–12 years post treatment. J Esthet Restor Dent 2002;14:275–285.

Rosenstiel SF, Gegauff AG, Johnson WM. Randomised clinical trial of the efficacy and safety of a home bleaching procedure. Quintessence Int 1996;27:413-424.

Russell CM, Dickinson GL, Johnson MH et al. Dentist-supervised home bleaching with ten per cent carbamide peroxide gel: a six month study. J Esthet Dent 1996;8:177–182.

Chapter 3

Management of Discoloured Dead Anterior Teeth

Aim

To consider relevant terminology and the methods of dealing with dead discoloured teeth, to describe the inside/outside bleaching technique in detail, and to consider alternative techniques and how to manage problems.

Outcome

The practitioner will be aware of predictable approaches to bleaching discoloured, dead anterior teeth and that bleaching is the most effective way of managing these teeth. The practitioner needs to be conscious of the destructive nature of alternative interventive treatments.

Discoloured Dead Teeth

Dentists often refer to dead teeth as *non-vital* teeth, and patients are frequently bemused by this. This is a good example of not using plain English! To most people the word vital means essential. In dental terms non-vital describes a tooth that has a dead pulp or has had the pulp removed as part of an endodontic procedure.

Patients with a low lip line may well accept a mildly discoloured dead front tooth while those with a high lip line may very well find any discolouration unacceptable. Such discolouration is often the reason for seeking treatment.

Improving the appearance of a discoloured dead front tooth can have a profound effect on the patient's self-confidence and oral health. Such thinking has been recognised by the World Health Organization, which has stated that "Health is a state of complete physical, mental and social well-being and not merely the absence of disease or infirmity" (1994). Marked discolouration of teeth can be a serious handicap which impacts on a person's self-image, self-confidence, physical attractiveness and employability.

Assessment

The successful management of discoloured dead teeth is based on an accurate diagnosis followed by detailed treatment planning. A comprehensive history should be taken, including details of events that may have contributed to the discolouration. A detailed clinical examination, including special investigations as indicated clinically, should then follow.

A focused approach will reduce the chances of overlooking critical information and avoid failure of treatment. Patient input is critical. A full and frank discussion of a patient's perceptions of their problem is especially important in assessing whether or not they have realistic expectations of the outcome of treatment. Whatever treatment plan is agreed, it should provide the best possible prospects for a durable, predictable, aesthetically pleasing and cost-effective result for the patient. This should be accomplished with the least possible biological damage.

Aetiology

The most common cause of discolouration in dead teeth is the presence of residual pulpal haemorrhagic products. These are most likely to be left in the pulp horn spaces and cervical region. The discolouration is usually caused by breakdown products of haemoglobin and other haematin molecules, which may permeate into the dentine of the dead tooth.

Trauma is the most common cause of dead front teeth. Patients may not give a clear history of the relevant trauma. They may have been under the influence of alcohol or drugs at the time or they may have been more concerned about other injuries and therefore overlooked the trauma to their teeth. The discolouration, which may be gradual, is often painless and may only become apparent when others comment on it. Discolouration of a dead tooth may be an incidental finding in a routine dental examination.

Discolouration often follows endodontic treatment of a tooth. Indeed, many patients on being told that they need a root filling ask if their tooth will turn black afterwards as a consequence of this.

About 10% of patients may be unhappy with the appearance of their root-filled teeth. Incorporating blood or other stain into the tooth/restoration interface may cause, or substantially contribute to, discolouration. Materials used in endodontic procedures, including root canal sealants containing silver, eugenol, polyantibiotic pastes, and compounds containing phenol, may cause darkening of the root dentine. Metallic points, pins and posts inserted into dead teeth are a frequent cause of discolouration. In addition, leakage of restorations may be a causative or contributing factor. Sadly, much of the discolouration seen in endodontically treated teeth can be described as iatrogenic. Figs 3-1 and 3-2 show upper incisors before and after bleaching.

Mechanisms of Discolouration

When teeth suffer significant trauma there is disruption of the pulp contents and vascularity. This can result in haemorrhage and subsequent tooth discolouration. The extent to which the products of pulp degradation contribute to tooth discolouration remains unclear. It is considered that pulpal ischaemia and subsequent pulp death, in the absence of bacterial contamination, does not produce discolouration to the same extent as overt haemorrhage into the pulp chamber. Following haemorrhage, the haemoglobin molecules may be found to be concentrated mainly in the coronal dentine close to the pulp. They do not tend to penetrate far into the dentinal tubules. This largely explains why inside/outside bleaching produces predictably satisfactory results.

In traumatised teeth marked changes in colour appear to occur only when there has been frank haemorrhage into the pulp chamber. The coloured pigment responsible for the discolouration arises from the haemoglobin in the red blood cells. The cementum layer appears to act as a barrier to the passage of the blood pigments, preventing root surfaces from being discoloured by blood from bleeding of the soft tissues.

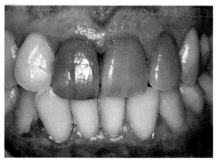 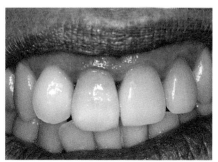

Fig 3-1 Discoloured upper incisors before bleaching.

Fig 3-2 Upper incisors after bleaching.

Any methods attempting to remove discolouration following trauma and haemorrhage into the pulp chamber should focus on the removal of the breakdown products of blood. The pulp chamber is surrounded by dentine and isolated from any inflammatory or healing response in the adjacent soft tissues. Therefore, normal healing, which could occur for example with a black eye, with the eventual loss of discolouration in the tissues, cannot occur. If the pulp does not survive following trauma and haemorrhage then the haematin material remains within the pulp chamber and consequently the tooth appears discoloured. On the other hand, if revascularisation occurs and the pulp survives then the tooth can revert to its normal colour within two to three months.

Monitoring

The colour of teeth can be monitored by using a shade guide or by taking photographs with a shade tab beside the tooth. A record should be kept. Follow-up reviews of root canal treatment should include a check for discolouration using the shade guide or photograph as a reference. If discolouration is observed, it is better to intervene sooner rather than later. Later discolouration may indicate, among other possibilities, leakage or degradation of the endodontic sealer. Delaying treatment may well result in the discolouration being more difficult to treat.

Inside/outside Bleaching

Prior to undertaking inside/outside bleaching the tooth should be root-filled in a standard fashion, under rubber dam using copious amounts of hypochlorite. Hypochlorite is a bleach and although mainly used as an antiseptic it inadvertently also removes some of the discolouration. However, this is not nearly as effective as the carbamide peroxide used in inside/outside bleaching.

This technique involves placing 10% carbamide peroxide gel simultaneously on and inside a discoloured root-filled tooth, usually with the aid of a single-tooth customised tray. This allows penetration of hydrogen peroxide both internally and externally, with the bleaching gel being protected from salivary deactivation by the tray (see Figs 3-3 to 3-5).

Access is gained to the pulp chamber via a standard access cavity (Fig 3-6, page 40). Prior to bleaching, the contents of the chamber should be removed and the chamber thoroughly cleaned for about five minutes with an ultrasonic tip (Fig 3-7). The root filling is reduced to a level below the

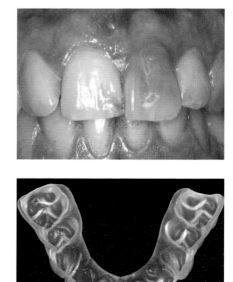

Fig 3-3 Discoloured luxated extruded upper left incisor.

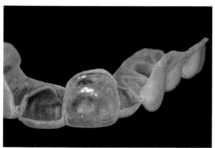

Fig 3-4 Single-tooth tray.

Fig 3-5 Occlusal view of single-tooth tray.

cemento–enamel junction and is usually sealed off with a radiopaque glass ionomer or zinc polycarboxylate cement. It is technically difficult to place this cement seal accurately. It is essential, however, that the cement does not contact the discoloured dentinal walls because if it does this will compromise effective bleaching of the neck of the tooth.

In cases of marked cervical discolouration it is possible to undertake bleaching without sealing over the root filling, provided patient cooperation is very good and the access cavity can be kept constantly bathed in 10% carbamide peroxide. Carbamide peroxide is a well-proven oxidising antiseptic and will inhibit Gram-negative anaerobic bacteria very effectively.

Any composite on the external or internal surfaces of the tooth must be removed before bleaching, as the hydrogen peroxide cannot penetrate through composite. The endodontic access cavity is left open for the duration of the inside/outside bleaching procedure, which usually takes two to four days.

39

The 10% carbamide peroxide gel, both within the tooth and in the tray, is changed every two hours and last thing at night. The more often the gel is changed, the quicker bleaching will occur.

The tray is worn continuously, except during eating, cleaning and replacing the gel. When changing the gel, and in particular after eating, the access cavity is flushed out using a syringe of the gel. Because of its viscous nature this syringing effect removes any food debris and ensures that the cavity is filled with fresh gel. The patient will not experience sensitivity because the tooth is root-filled.

The patient is instructed to stop bleaching when they are satisfied with the degree of lightening of the tooth. It is acceptable for the tooth to go a little lighter to allow for "rebound" of the colour. The patient is reviewed after two to three days to assess colour changes and to limit the time the access cavity is left open (see Figs 3-6 to 3-13).

It is not unusual for patients to get excited and to telephone the practice to say that the tooth has changed its colour after only 24 hours. Such cases may be reviewed sooner than planned but it is generally prudent to suggest continuing bleaching for two to three days.

Following successful completion of bleaching, the pulp chamber is once again thoroughly cleaned with the aid of an ultrasonic tip. The tooth is provisionally restored with a glass ionomer cement.

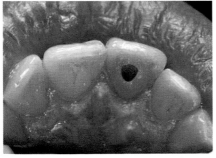

Fig 3-6 Mirror view of upper left central incisor showing access cavity.

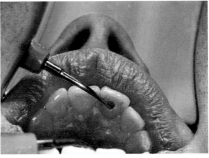

Fig 3-7 Ultrasonic cleaning of the chamber to below the cemento–enamel junction.

During the bleaching procedure, contamination of the root canal system by highly colorific materials should be avoided. Patients need to be advised to avoid foods such as curries, tomato-containing sauces and dark-coloured

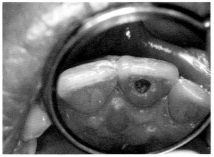

Fig 3-8 Gutta-percha cut back below the cemento–enamel junction.

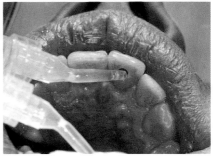

Fig 3-9 Patient injecting 10% carbamide peroxide into the tooth.

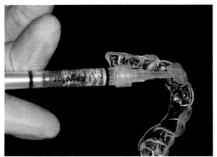

Fig 3-10 Tray being loaded with 10% carbamide peroxide.

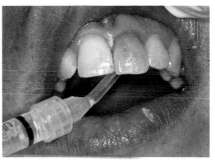

Fig 3-11 Colour change at 24 hours.

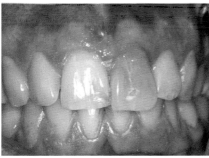

Fig 3-12 Upper left central incisor before treatment.

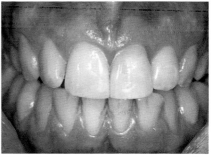

Fig 3-13 Upper left central incisor after treatment. (It has also been shortened.)

fluids until the access cavity is restored. They should be advised to avoid drinking red wine, coffee or strong tea until such time as the tooth has been definitively sealed.

Following bleaching, the tooth frequently appears to be lighter than the adjacent tooth. This is understandable given the reduction in the volume of dentine within the root-filled tooth.

A composite restoration should not be placed immediately following completion of the bleaching process because oxygen will be released from the tooth for up to a week. This could compromise the composite bond and thereby lead to leakage (see Figs 3-14 and 3-15).

The central part of the tooth should be restored with a material having shade and optical properties similar to intact dentine. As composites are notoriously difficult to remove from within the tooth without inadvertently removing residual tooth structure, there are benefits in selecting a glass ionomer cement to replace lost dentine. It is possible to check that the appearance of the restored tooth will be acceptable by leaving some water inside the access cavity and placing the selected material on a trial basis to check that it will achieve the desired outcome. A trial assessment of the colour done in this way is infinitely preferable to having to drill out a definitive set restoration which fails to achieve the desired outcome.

If there is any concern about the endodontic status, the tooth should be re-root-filled prior to commencing inside/outside bleaching.

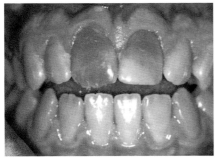

Fig 3-14 Dead upper central incisors with composite on the tip of the upper left central incisor.

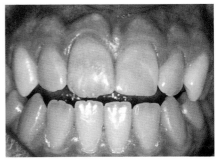

Fig 3-15 Composite replaced one week after bleaching.

Protocol for Inside/outside Bleaching

First Appointment

1. Make and record the diagnosis.
2. Take a photograph.
3. Check the periapical status of the tooth with a long cone periapical radiograph. Be satisfied that the root space is satisfactorily obturated.
4. Undertake any necessary endodontic revision prior to starting inside/outside bleaching.
5. Check that the tooth is asymptomatic and has a favourable prognosis.
6. Use a shade guide to estimate the shade before treatment. Agree the shade with the patient, record it in the clinical records and give the patient a copy.
7. Warn the patient that any existing matching restorations within the target and adjacent teeth will not bleach. After bleaching, such restorations may well appear to be darker than the bleached tooth. Consequently, the restorations may need to be replaced. In all such cases the patient should be warned of this aesthetic and financial consequence of bleaching.
8. A diagram of the existing restorations is made and given to the patient, with a copy being kept in the clinical records.
9. Discuss other treatment options, highlighting the minimally invasive nature of bleaching.
10. Check that the patient is not allergic to peroxide or plastic and that female patients of child-bearing age are not pregnant or breastfeeding.
11. Provide the patient with a written treatment plan and estimates and obtain consent.
12. Provide the patient with written instructions and demonstrate what the treatment involves.
13. Make contemporaneous notes that this protocol has been completed.

Making the Tray

An alginate impression is taken and cast in the laboratory. Proprietary resin, or failing that plaster, is used to block out the cast on the **labial and palatal** aspects of the target tooth. The blocking out should provide the desired extent and depth of the intended reservoirs.

Cold-mould seal is applied to the cast. Softened bleaching-tray material is then vacuum-formed to the cast and, once cooled, removed. Labial windows are cut out over the adjacent teeth so that only the target tooth is covered. Any gel that strays on to the adjacent teeth will be inactivated by the saliva. In this way only the target tooth will be bleached.

Second Appointment

1. Check the bleaching tray for fit and comfort and that the patient is able to place and remove it.

2. Remove the access cavity restoration and reduce the root filling as necessary to a level 2 mm below the cemento–enamel junction. A fine ultrasonic tip is the simplest way to do this. The root filling is then sealed, taking care not to put any sealing material on the discoloured dentinal walls. A radiopaque glass ionomer cement is ideal for this purpose. It should be allowed time to set fully.

   If any sealing material is placed over the discoloured dentine, it will effectively stop the bleach from working in that area. The result is frequently a disappointing appearance, following the consequent failure to bleach the neck of the tooth. The worry about disruption of the root filling and a theoretic bacterial recontamination of the root filling needs to be weighed against the requirement to achieve a good aesthetic result. In weighing up the risks of the treatment, it should be remembered that failure to bleach the neck of the tooth may necessitate having to resort to a very destructive interventive procedure, including the possible provision of a post crown.

3. The pulp chamber is checked for any residual debris and root canal material. This is critical to the procedure. The pulp cornuae and the cervical region are cleaned ultrasonically for at least five minutes.

   It is prudent to "check etch" the inside of the tooth to see if all the exposed dentine takes on a cleaned appearance, indicating that the surfaces have been properly prepared and are free of any residual tooth-coloured filling material – in particular, composite. Any composite on the labial aspect of the tooth should be removed. The outside of the tooth should also be etched with phosphoric acid. A frosty appearance will confirm that the enamel is free of resin tags.

4. The 10% carbamide peroxide gel is injected directly into the chamber of the tooth. The tray, with gel in the target teeth reservoirs only, is inserted into the mouth. Excess gel is wiped away with gauze.

5. Provide the patient with enough of the appropriate gel and written instructions. Demonstrate what to do. Check that the patient can insert the gel effectively into the tooth using the syringe and angled needle tip.

6. If the patient is unable to place the gel effectively, an immediate fallback position is for the dentist to seal some carbamide peroxide in the pulp chamber and have the patient use the bleaching tray to carry out external bleaching. However, this is not as effective as inside/outside bleaching.

Instructions for Patients

1. Remove the top from the syringe containing the 10% carbamide peroxide gel. Screw a blunt standard right-angled needle tip onto the syringe. Insert the tip of the needle into the cavity on the inside of the tooth to be bleached and fill the cavity within the tooth with the gel.
2. Load the appropriate part of the bleaching tray with the 10% carbamide peroxide gel. (A mark made on the outside of the tray with a permanent ink pen may help identify that part of the tray to be loaded with the gel.)
3. Insert the tray and remove any excess gel with a finger or a soft toothbrush.
4. Rinse the mouth gently with water and spit out.
5. Wear the tray at all times, except when eating or cleaning.
6. Every 2 hours and last thing at night change the gel inside the tooth and also in the tray. Clean the inside of the tooth by flushing it out with the bleaching gel.
7. The tray can be cleaned with water and a toothbrush.
8. Avoid highly coloured foods such as curries, tomato-containing sauces and dark-coloured fruits. Red wine, coffee and strong tea must be avoided until bleaching has been completed and the tooth is sealed by the placement of a filling.
9. If there are any problems contact the practice immediately.
10. Stop bleaching when the tooth is the desired colour.

Problems and Troubleshooting

Poor Patient Compliance

Good patient selection and clear instructions should minimise this problem. Inability, or unwillingness, to follow the instructions will lead to failure or prolonged treatment time. The patient must understand their responsibilities and role in their treatment. Inside/outside bleaching should not be undertaken when a patient is not well known to the practitioner.

The patient has to have reasonable manual dexterity and must be able to place the gel within the tooth. This can be checked before making the tray and opening the access cavity by testing whether the patient is able to hold the syringe effectively against the inside of the tooth. If the patient is unable or unwilling to do this, then alternative treatment options should be considered.

Patients may sometimes complain about food getting into the access cavity. This should not create any great difficulty, assuming the patient is properly briefed and capable of placing and using the bleaching gel syringe to flush out any food debris.

The Neck of the Tooth Does not Bleach

This is typically caused by restoration material being still bonded to the inside of the tooth. Hydrogen peroxide cannot penetrate through any residual cement or resin. Magnification should be used to ensure complete and safe removal of all materials covering the dentine to be bleached. It is prudent to "check etch" the inside of the tooth. Dentine with a frosted appearance indicates that its surface is free of residual tooth-coloured materials.

Failure to reduce the root filling to a level well below the cemento–enamel junction will hinder the penetration of the bleaching agent into the dentine forming the neck of the tooth. Furthermore, the tray needs to be extended cervically to cover the gingival margin to hold the bleaching gel in and around the cervical region. Enamel is thin in the cervical region and therefore it is important that the underlying discoloured dentine is adequately bleached. The needle on the syringe helps ensure that the gel is placed into the deepest part of the tooth.

Failure to Bleach

If the tooth fails to bleach despite appropriate clinical technique and good patient compliance, the source of the discolouration is probably not pulpal in origin. A history of an amalgam restoration in the palatal access cavity is frequently the cause. Metal ions, which migrate from the amalgam into the adjacent tooth structure, are much more resistant to bleaching than the discolouring molecules that originate from the pulp. If any amalgam is left in the tooth during bleaching, the tooth may take on a green tinge. It is therefore essential to remove all amalgam from within the tooth before undertaking inside/outside bleaching (Figs 3-16 and 3-17).

The presence of a labial porcelain veneer means that the reservoir must be placed on the palatal aspect as the porcelain is impervious to the hydrogen peroxide. With this approach the tooth can be bleached successfully without removing the porcelain veneer.

Fig 3-16 A dead root-filled tooth with a porcelain veneer but without the contents of the pulp chamber having been removed. Sealing the access cavity with amalgam made this problem worse. Tarnish and corrosion products from the silver of the amalgam have contributed to the discolouration.

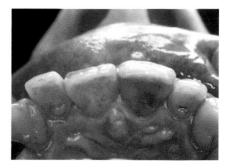

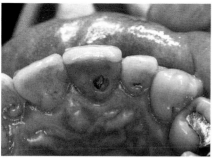

Fig 3-17 Amalgam removed before inside/outside bleaching.

Fig 3-18 Bocasan is a source of sodium perborate.

Discolouration Difficult to Manage

Where a tooth has been discoloured, for example by tetracycline therapy and trauma, then the combination of discolouration may be difficult to manage. The various options are discussed below.

"Walking bleach"

This technique involves the use of a mixture of water and sodium perborate (Fig 3-18) which is sealed temporarily into the pulp chamber of the dead root-filled tooth.

The difficulty with this treatment is that the continual bubbling of the oxygen being released from the hydrogen peroxide very frequently "blows" the temporary dressing out of the back of the tooth. In addition, the wet environment, caused by the continual bubbling of the bleaching paste, makes it very difficult to reseal the tooth. As a result, the hydrogen peroxide may not be contained adequately in the tooth long enough to bleach the dentine.

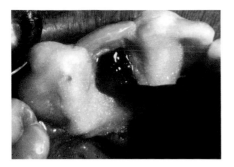

Fig 3-19 Application of 38% hydrogen peroxide with Opaldam (Ultradent Products Inc.).

Chair-side bleaching
Chair-side bleaching involves the use of high-concentration (30–38%) hydrogen peroxide, sometimes together with heat applied both inside and outside the tooth. This technique involves the use of a material which is about 10 times the strength of hydrogen peroxide released from 10% carbamide peroxide (Fig 3-19).

Rubber dam or a light cured dam must be used, given the caustic nature of the bleaching agent.

If this approach is used inside the tooth, the root filling must be carefully sealed off and care taken to avoid penetration of the bleaching gel through to the periodontal ligament. The high-concentration hydrogen peroxide used may damage the periodontal ligament, compromising the clinical outcome. About 2% of teeth have a defect at the cemento–enamel junction and very high-concentration material may damage the periodontal ligament if it leaches out in that area. If this happens, invasive cervical resorption can occur but this has been reported only when high concentrations (30-38%) hydrogen peroxide have been used in conjunction with heat (Fig 3-20).

Resorption has **never** been reported using 10% carbamide peroxide with the inside/outside technique.

Removal of the access cavity restoration gives access to the contents of the pulp chamber. Thorough ultrasonic cleaning with a fine tip will remove a substantial amount of discoloured material by eliminating any residual pulpal remnants and any material which may have accumulated in the pulp space through leakage.

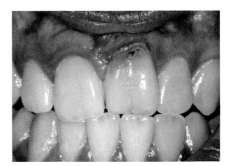

Fig 3-20 Resorption of the upper left central incisor following trauma, late reimplantation and chair-side bleaching.

Restorative Options

Porcelain or composite veneers

The placement of a veneer on a deeply discoloured front tooth will not provide a satisfactory result. The underlying discolouration is often most noticeable in the cervical region where there is very little, if any, enamel to conceal the underlying dentine and the veneer has to be at its thinnest in that area. To mask the discolouration it may be necessary to produce a thick over-contoured veneer, including an opaque layer, which compromises the appearance of the veneer. Excessive reduction of the tooth exposes a significant amount of discoloured dentine. It is common to find that discolouration gets worse the deeper the preparation because dark dentine in the cervical region is no longer masked by enamel. The darkest dentine is nearest the pulp space.

A thick opaque veneer placed on a discoloured tooth will not match the adjacent translucent teeth. The life expectancy of a thick veneer bonded to deep, discoloured dentine is uncertain. What is clear is that once the patient has had a veneer, the tooth will have been weakened and the veneer will require a lifetime of maintenance, with the possibility of the further loss of tooth tissue as and when the veneer may need to be replaced.

Crowns and post crowns

Preparations for crowns are very destructive of the remaining tooth tissue. Preparation of a root-filled tooth for a conventional crown often results in a post being necessary to support a replacement core. Such an approach does not address the discolouration within the remaining root dentine. Gingival recession frequently exposes the margin of the crown and the discoloured root dentine. This is especially likely in a young patient when full maturation of the gingival tissues is likely to result in an unsightly gingival appearance.

49

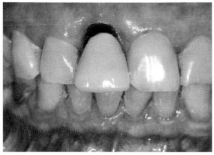

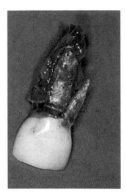

Fig 3-21 Gingival recession exposes the dark root.

Fig 3-22 Fractured root caused by post crown (following extraction).

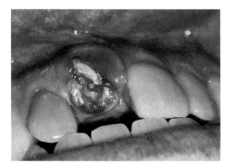

Fig 3-23 Fractured root in position. The upper right lateral incisor although dead is still structurally intact and suitable for inside/outside bleaching.

This is sometimes unkindly called the "Neapolitan ice-cream effect" with the transition from white (the artificial crown) to brown/black (the root) and then the pink of the receded gingival tissues (Fig 3-21).

The aesthetic difficulties associated with the provision of a single anterior crown, in particular a post crown, are well known. An aggressive crown approach to the management of discoloured dead teeth greatly weakens the remaining tooth tissues, is costly and may result in catastrophic failure sooner or later. Recent developments in tooth-coloured resin bonded post systems have not overcome all the inherent structural strength disadvantages of the post crown approach to dealing with these aesthetic problems (Figs 3-22 and 3-23).

Inside/outside bleaching has dramatically reduced the incidence of root fractures by post crowns. It removes the discolouration while maintaining the structure of the tooth. This is particularly important when a high lip line exposes the gingival margins (Figs 3-24 and 3-25).

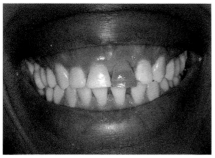 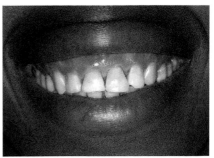

Fig 3-24 Before inside/outside bleaching.   **Fig 3-25** After inside/outside bleaching.

Summary of the Management of Discoloured Dead Anterior Teeth

Monitor and review
Inside/outside bleaching technique with 10% carbamide peroxide
Walking bleach technique Just using carbamide peroxide which releases 3.5% hydrogen peroxide Sodium perborate and water which releases 7% hydrogen peroxide Sodium perborate and 18% hydrogen peroxide which releases about 25% hydrogen peroxide
External bleaching Chair-side bleaching or home bleaching or a combination of both. Chair-side bleaching using heat and a high concentration (30-38%) of hydrogen peroxide (**highest risk of resorption**)
Restorative techniques
Veneers – direct composites Veneers – indirect composites Porcelain veneers Crown, with or without a post Extraction and prosthetic replacement

Least destructive → Most destructive

Further Reading

Baldwin DC. Appearance and aesthetics in oral health. Community Dent Oral Epidemiol 1980;8:244–256.

Haywood VB, Heymann HO. Nightguard vital bleaching. Quintessence Int 1989;20:173–176.

Heithersay GS. Invasive cervical resorption: an analysis of potential predisposing factors. Quintessence Int 1999;30:83–95.

Nutting EB, Poe GS. Chemical bleaching of discolored endodontically treated teeth. Dent Clin North Am 1967; 655–662.

Poyser NJ, Kelleher MG, Briggs PF. Managing discoloured non-vital teeth: the inside/outside bleaching technique. Dental Update 2004;May:204–210:213–214.

Settembrini L, Gultz J, Kaim J, Scherer W. A technique for bleaching non-vital teeth: inside/outside bleaching. J Am Dent Assoc 1997;128:1283–1284.

Spasser HF. A simple bleaching technique using sodium perborate. New York State Dent J 1961;27:332–334.

World Health Organization Oral Health. Oral Health for the 21st Century. Geneva: WHO,1994.

Chapter 4
Bleaching of Teeth Affected by Specific Conditions

Aim

The aim is to discuss the bleaching of teeth discoloured by fluorosis, tetracyclines and certain congenital problems.

Outcome

The practitioner will be aware of the causes of atypical discolouration and of the various bleaching techniques that can be used in their management.

Introduction

Correct diagnosis of the causes of discolouration is essential in its management. Other causes of discolouration are detailed in Chapter 7.

Fluorosis

Fluorosis causes brown spots or white flecks on teeth. The appearance varies from white striations or localised spots to yellow or brown bands or general discolouration of enamel, with or without pits and other surface abnormalities (Figs 4-1 and 4-2).

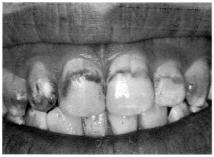

Fig 4-1 Brown and white fluorosis.

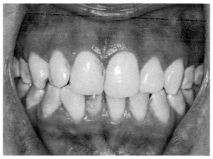

Fig 4-2 Appearance after three weeks of nightguard vital bleaching with 10% carbamide peroxide.

In moderate fluorosis there is subsurface porosity which typically appears to resemble white spot lesions.

In more severe fluorosis there is pitting and loss of the outer layer of enamel, increasing the risk of caries through plaque accumulation and retention.

Appearance of Fluorosis
Fluorosis is often first seen in the gingival third of the second primary molars. This presentation is usually indicative of fluorosis being a problem for at least the permanent anterior teeth.

Classically, the banding type of fluorosis follows the developmental lines of the enamel and is symmetrical. Because mild white fluorosis is common and is of little, if any, clinical consequence, some dentists regard this as acceptable and a small price to pay for a substantial reduction in caries.

Cause of Fluorosis
Fluorosis is caused by exposure to too much fluoride during the development of the dentition. The main risks for developing fluorosis are swallowing toothpaste, excessive fluoride supplements and baby food reconstituted with fluoridated water (Figs 4-3 and 4-4).

Swallowing Toothpaste
The aesthetic damage caused by fluorosis is often done before a child sees a dentist. A lot of fluorosis is related to unsupervised tooth brushing with relatively large amounts of toothpaste with the toothpaste being swallowed rather than being spat out. Over 90% of toothpastes contain fluoride, usually with 1450 parts per million (ppm). Flavoured toothpastes have been shown to be associated with an increased use of toothpaste by children.

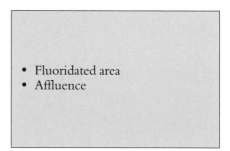

- The age that brushing commences
- The frequency of brushing
- The fluoride concentration i.e. 650 ppm vs 1450 ppm
- The amount of toothpaste applied to the brush and subsequently swallowed

- Fluoridated area
- Affluence

Fig 4-3 Risk factors for developing fluorosis from toothbrushing.

Fig 4-4 General risk factors.

Summary

- Parents should be encouraged to supervise tooth brushing
- Use small amounts of children's toothpaste
- Encourage the spitting out of waste slurry
- The use of toothpastes containing low concentrations of fluoride is appropriate for:
  - children at low risk of caries
  - children living in a fluoridated area
  - children living in areas of relative affluence

Fig 4-5 Preventing fluorosis.

The higher the socio-economic group the greater the use of toothpaste. Toothpastes for children with lower concentrations of fluoride (e.g. 650 ppm) are available but many families, for convenience and through lack of awareness, just use one regular toothpaste for all the family. However, the use of toothpastes with lower fluoride content (650 ppm) may reduce protection against possible development of caries in susceptible children.

Young children swallow between half and 90% of toothpaste used. They should be supervised when brushing and only small amounts of toothpaste should be used. Toothpaste should be applied across the brush rather than along it as this limits the amount used more effectively. Children should spit out used toothpaste but not rinse. In this way the teeth are bathed in fluoride for some time and this helps reduce the risk of caries (Fig 4-5).

Management of Fluorosis
Nightguard vital bleaching is the treatment of choice. Localised brown fluorosis located well away from the gingival margin can be dealt with by careful chair-side bleaching. Bleaching should be undertaken before resorting to any invasive procedure such as microabrasion. Microabrasion should precede direct bonding with composite. Porcelain veneers should be a last resort given the loss of enamel necessary to achieve a satisfactory aesthetic outcome.

Brown fluorotic spots respond moderately well to bleaching. White flecks are usually less obvious or worrying than brown ones but can look more obvious during the bleaching process, when the teeth affected become "blotchy". This is not normally a problem once the bleaching has been completed as the white flecks are less obvious against the lightened background. This is usually acceptable to most patients.

Protocol for Bleaching Fluorotic Teeth

1. Identify the areas of fluorosis and record them in the dental notes. Take photographs and discuss the treatment options. Warn about secondary flecking (white fluorotic flecks on teeth) which patients or parents usually do not notice until the brown fluorosis (Fig 4-6) has been bleached away.
2. Dry the teeth and apply a contrasting coloured (old or scarcely used) composite over the brown areas without etching the teeth (Fig 4-7).
3. Light-cure this composite in position (Fig 4-8).
4. Take an impression with the composite still on the teeth.
5. Remove the composite from the teeth.
6. When the impression is cast, the teeth will appear overbuilt in the areas of maximum discolouration (Fig 4-9).
7. Once formed, the tray will have reservoirs corresponding to where the composite was applied (Fig 4-10). This allows the gel to be held in the tray over the areas selected for bleaching.
8. The tray is cut back to produce windows as appropriate (Fig 4-10). Teeth that are not being bleached will be bathed in saliva and this prevents them from being bleached.
9. The patient is shown how to put the 10% carbamide peroxide in the tray. The patient is told to wear this every night until happy with the colour change (Figs 4-11 and 4-12).

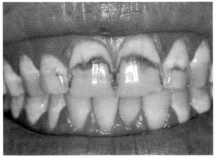

Fig 4-6 Brown banded fluorosis.

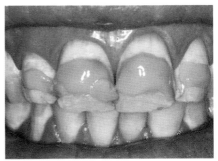

Fig 4-7 Composite applied over the dried, *not etched,* brown areas.

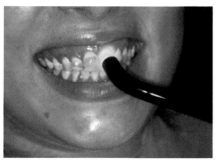

Fig 4-8 Composite being light-cured.

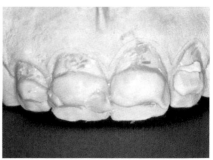

Fig 4-9 Positive areas on the cast.

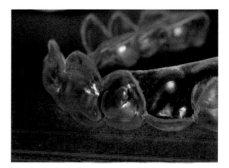

Fig 4-10 Reservoirs correspond to where the composite was placed on teeth. Windows are cut over teeth not to be bleached.

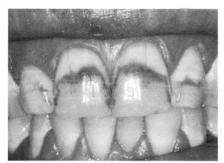

Fig 4-11 Teeth with banded fluorosis.

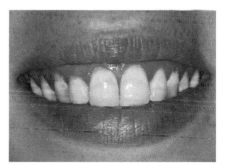

Fig 4-12 Teeth following four weeks of nightguard vital bleaching with 10% carbamide peroxide.

Treatment Times

There are no particular reasons for delaying the bleaching of fluorosed teeth. Bleaching is safe in young patients and can be undertaken as soon as the first permanent molars are sufficiently erupted to retain the tray for conventional nightguard vital bleaching with 10% carbamide peroxide. This can be started as soon as a tray can be tolerated and retained in position by the child.

Chair-side bleaching using up to 38% hydrogen peroxide can be undertaken in young patients, but only if there is excellent cooperation and if effective isolation can be achieved. Localised small brown areas of fluorosis, usually well away from the gingival margin, can be successfully bleached using this technique.

Bleaching of moderately fluorosed teeth takes about four to six weeks to complete. A review at about one month is generally indicated. Bleaching may be safely extended over a period of at least six months but this is rarely necessary in the management of fluorosis.

Mild sensitivity is a common complaint but this typically resolves in a few days after bleaching has stopped. In the event of sensitivity developing before bleaching is completed the bleaching regimen may be changed to every second night rather than every night. This approach is a compromise which delays the bleaching process but will achieve a good result.

To reduce sensitivity, toothpaste containing 5% potassium nitrate (KNO_3) can be placed in the bleaching tray, which can be worn for half an hour prior to bleaching. This toothpaste needs to be washed out of the tray before inserting the 10% carbamide peroxide. This technique reduces sensitivity and improves patient compliance and satisfaction with the bleaching process.

Figs 4-13 shows brown fluorosis in a young teenager and Figs 4-14 and 4-15 show the teenager before and after bleaching.

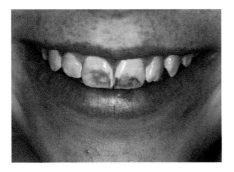

Fig 4-13 Marked brown fluorosis in a young teenager.

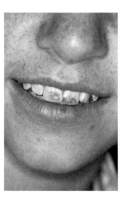

Fig 4-14
View of a
young
teenager with
brown
fluorosis.

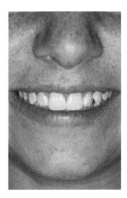

Fig 4-15
View follow-
ing bleaching.

Troubleshooting

Where there is a mixture of brown fluorosis and white fluorotic flecks ("secondary flecking") it is important to draw attention to the less obvious white fluorosis. Patients and their parents should be warned that the brown fluorosis is likely to reduce gradually in a blotchy pattern. They should be reassured when this pattern becomes obvious and advised to carry on bleaching. As bleaching progresses, the white flecks, while still present and evident on close examination, are usually less obvious against the bleached background.

Fig 4-16 shows brown and white fluorosis before bleaching and Fig 4-17 shows the appearance following poor-compliance bleaching.

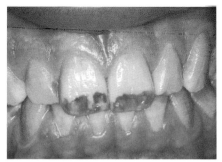

Fig 4-16 Brown and white fluorosis before bleaching.

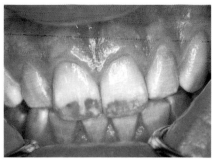

Fig 4-17 Appearance after poor compliance and only intermittent use of nightguard bleaching with 10% carbamide peroxide.

Microabrasion

The simplest way to effect microabrasion of recalcitrant flourotic areas is to use a fine multibladed tungsten carbide bur (Jet FG 7901) held in a high-speed handpiece and operated with a feather-light touch (Fig 4-18). Microabrasion should be undertaken only following prolonged nightguard vital bleaching extending over at least two months.

Any form of destructive removal of enamel is to be avoided unless absolutely necessary. It is essential to warn the patient that enamel will be removed, is irreplaceable and that the discolouration may not be limited to the superficial layer to be reduced by microabrasion. Consent for microabrasion should be obtained from the patient prior to commencing treatment.

Microabrasion can be achieved with composite finishing discs but this technique results in a generalised flattening of the enamel surface. Alternatively, microabrasion can be undertaken using a slurry of 18% hydrochloric acid and pumice applied using a polishing cup operating at slow speed. This procedure must be undertaken under rubber dam as the slurry is acidic and splatter needs to be carefully controlled. Eye protection is essential for the patient, nurse and operator. The material of choice is Opalustre (Ultradent Products Inc.) (see Fig 4-19).

Microabrasion results in a ground glass effect termed *abrosion*, a term coined from abrasion and erosion (see Figs 4-20 and 4-21).

The most successful management of fluorosis is nightguard vital bleaching for as long as it takes (Figs 4-22 and 4-23). If there is a residual problem then use a conservative direct composite bonding technique rather than destroying the enamel surface. Given sufficient time even severe mottling

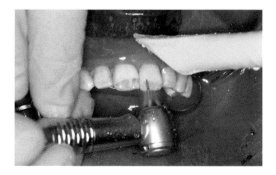

Fig 4-18 Microabrasion with a fine multibladed tungsten carbide bur.

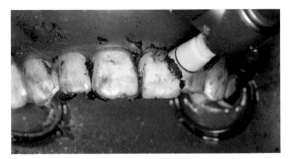

Fig 4-19 Microabrasion under rubber dam with 18% hydrochloric acid and pumice.

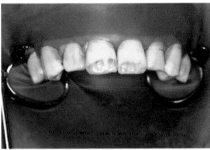

Fig 4-20 "Abrosion" immediately following treatment.

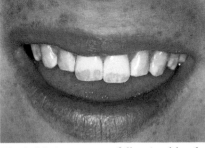

Fig 4-21 Appearance following bleaching and microabrasion (compare with Fig 4-16).

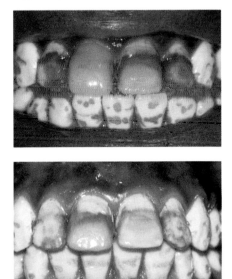

Fig 4-22 Teeth with endemic fluorosis.

Fig 4-23 Appearance following removal of composite and three months of intermittent bleaching with 10% carbamide peroxide. The teeth were sensitive despite the bleaching being limited to every second day for two hours only.

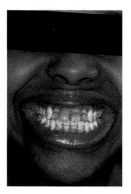

Fig 4-24
Teeth prior to bleaching.

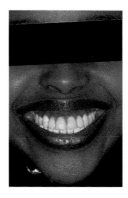

Fig 4-25
Following four months of bleaching the appearance of the bleached teeth was enhanced with direct composite.

will improve to the extent that simple direct composite bonding will achieve a favourable result (Figs 4-24 and 4-25).

Tetracycline Discolouration

Tetracyclines are broad spectrum antibiotics used in the treatment of a variety of infections, including acne, bronchitis, brucella, chlamydia and diseases caused by rickettsia (Q fever). They are widely used for respiratory diseases and in the management of genito-mycoplasma infections.

Tetracycline discolouration can be localised or generalised and often presents as horizontal banding. The banding relates to the time and duration of the ingestion of tetracycline, and when this occurred in relation to the time of the specific tooth development.

Minocycline hydrochloride is a broad spectrum antibiotic. It is widely used in the treatment of severe acne vulgaris (common acne). Minocycline has also been associated with the discolouration of teeth, bone, thyroid tissue and nails in young patients. Skin pigmentation may occur, particularly in relation to scar tissue. Ingestion of minocycline can produce discolouration in fully formed erupted teeth. The presence of discoloured bone may show through thin gingival tissues.

Tetracyclines have a very limited role in the treatment of acute oral infections as many causative organisms are resistant. Tetracyclines may have a role in the treatment of refractory forms of periodontal disease.

Mechanisms of Discolouration with Tetrocyclines

It has been recognised for many years that the deposition of tetracycline in growing bones and developing teeth causes discolouration by binding to calcium. Consequently tetracyclines should be avoided in the treatment of children under 12 years of age and women who are pregnant or breastfeeding.

The traditional explanation of the mechanism of tooth discolouration by tetracyclines is that they chelate or bind with calcium and iron during tooth development. Once the tetracycline molecule has bonded with calcium it is deposited at the predentine interface. It is then incorporated into the hydroxyapatite as a stable calcium orthophosphate compound. Exposure to ultraviolet light subsequent to eruption causes the initial yellow/brown fluorescence to change, probably through photo-oxidation. The result is a stable purple/red material 4, 12-anhydro-4-oxo-4-dedimethylaminotetracycline which causes tetracycline discoloured teeth to become darker. This change in discolouration is typically from yellow to brown. The brown appearance is caused by a mixture of unchanged yellow tetracycline orthophosphate and the purple-red of 4, 12-anhydro-4-oxo-4-dedimethylaminotetracyline.

Breakdown of Tetracyclines

Hydrogen peroxide eventually breaks down the stable ring structures, the quinonold chromophore, in the tetracycline molecules which cause tooth discolouration. These stable ring structures have double bonds which have to be broken into consecutive conjugated double bonds first and then into single bonds in order to result in lightening of the discoloured teeth. Tetracycline discolouration is only in the dentine and it is very stable. Bleaching of these teeth is slow and time-consuming.

Clinical Presentations

The presentation of tetracycline discolouration depends on the type of tetracycline which has been taken (Table 4-1). Other variables include the

Table 4-1 **Discolouration caused by different types of tetracycline**

Colour	Cause
Grey/brown	Chlortetracycline
Yellow/yellow brown	Demethylchlortetracycline
Brown/yellow	Oxytetracyline
Blue-grey/grey	Minocycline

age of the patient when the tetracycline was taken, the duration of the tetracycline treatment and the presence or absence of other conditions which may adversely affect tooth development. Figs 4-26 to 4-30 show different discolourations.

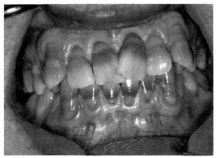

Fig 4-26 Tetracycline banding with crowding.

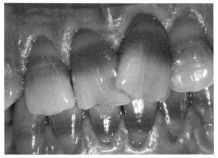

Fig 4-27 Mixed banded tetracycline discolouration. *Cervical*: demethylchlortetracycline; *middle:* oxytetracycline and chlortetracycline; *incisal:* chlortetracycline.

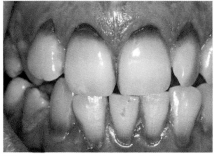

Fig 4-28 Cervical band of chlortetracycline discolouration.

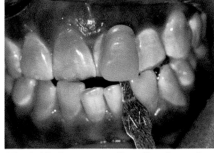

Fig 4-29 Oxytetracycline discolouration with shade tab in position as reference.

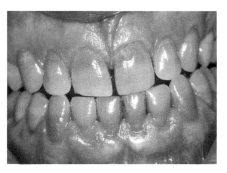

Fig 4-30 Chlortetracycline discolouration.

Bleaching vs Conventional Prosthodontics for Tetracycline Discolouration
Figs 4-31 to 4-36 show two contrasting approaches to the treatment of the same tetracycline discolouration in the same patient. The teeth in the lower arch were bleached with nightguard vital bleaching with 10% carbamide peroxide over a six-month period. The upper arch was treated with conventional full coverage crowns culminating in the loss of three teeth and the death of the upper right canine.

The upper right canine, root filled and with a post in it, is now vulnerable to a root fracture. Recession at the upper left central incisor and canine shows the dark roots. Bone resorption following the extraction of the upper right central and lateral incisors makes implants in this area impossible without bone grafting.

The patient gave a history of having had his discoloured teeth crowned around the age of 16 by a former dentist. He subsequently had severe toothache which led to root fillings, fractured crowns, replacement crowns, repeated infections and eventually to extractions. Following a period with a partial denture he had bridgework undertaken by another dentist in spite of the angulation difficulties. Subsequently the upper right canine was resected from the bridgework and restored with a separate post and crown leaving two units cantilevered from the abutments at the upper left central incisor and canine. Future bridgework on these three teeth would be even more unpredictable.

In contrast, the bleaching of the lower arch took six months with nightguard vital bleaching with 10% carbamide peroxide and the teeth are still structurally sound. The pulps have not been endangered in any way by this prolonged bleaching.

When concern is expressed about the effects of prolonged bleaching on pulps it should be noted that there have been no reports of pulpal death as a result of using 10% carbamide peroxide for even six to nine months. This is in marked contrast to the preparation for full-coverage restorations being associated with a one in six chance of pulpal death of the prepared teeth.

Differential Diagnosis
The nature of the discolouration of the teeth together with a history of tetracycline therapy is usually diagnostic of tetracycline discolouration. Other causes of discolouration, as discussed in Chapter 7, may need to be eliminated.

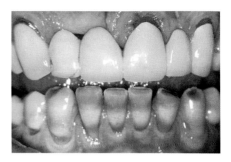

Fig 4-31 Upper teeth with conventional bridge and crown and lower teeth before bleaching.

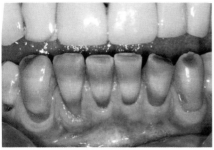

Fig 4-32 Lower teeth before bleaching.

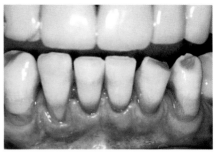

Fig 4-33 Lower teeth after bleaching.

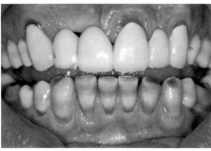

Fig 4-34 Teeth before bleaching.

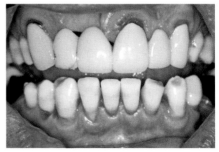

Fig 4-35 Teeth after bleaching.

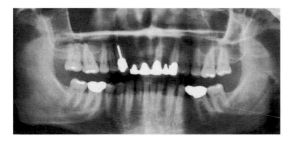

Fig 4-36 Radiograph showing upper bridge and post crown at the upper right canine.

Prevention
Healthcare professionals need to be aware of the discolouration of teeth caused by tetracyclines and to avoid prescribing these drugs to children under 12 years of age and women who are pregnant or breastfeeding.

Patients with a history of acne vulgaris (common acne) may have been prescribed minocycline for this. This drug can affect even fully formed erupted teeth but any such discoloured teeth can be effectively bleached with nightguard vital bleaching.

Treatment Protocol
Tetracycline discolouration is notoriously tedious to bleach. It is possible to achieve successful clinical outcomes using nightguard bleaching with 10% carbamide peroxide over prolonged periods of time. This is a safe and proven method with no adverse reactions having been reported in active treatments extending over periods of up to nine months.

Banded Tetracycline Discolouration
In treating banded tetracycline discolouration it is important to place the bleaching gel in the reservoirs which should be placed over the most intense areas of discolouration. To make a tray with accurately located reservoirs, composite can be used (see Figs 4-37 to 4-41). The teeth are dried but not etched and the composite is placed just where the teeth are most discoloured. The composite is cured and an impression taken. After the impression has been taken the composite is removed from the teeth with a flat plastic instrument. Care should be taken to ensure that the composite does not adhere to the tooth surface where the surface is rough or the enamel has lost its gloss. Replicas of the composite will appear as positive excesses on the model.

When the warmed clear thermoplastic material is blown down on the trimmed cast the positive excesses will produce the reservoirs where the bleaching gel needs to be in order to be at its most effective (Fig 4-42).

Figs 4-43 to 4-45 show the clinical appearance and the results of bleaching.

Efficacy
Follow-up reviews indicate that tetracycline discoloured teeth can be successfully bleached with the shade achieved being stable for periods of up to seven years. Patients are very positive about the benefits of the treatment and the lack of side-effects.

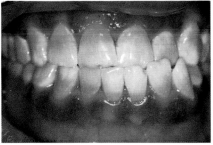

Fig 4-37 Cervical oxytetracycline discolouration. Note the cross bite.

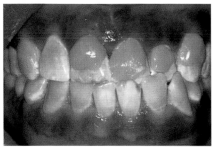

Fig 4-38 Composite applied to dried, but not etched, tooth surfaces over the darkest areas where the reservoirs are required.

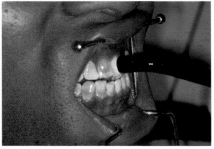

Fig 4-39 Composite cured in position.

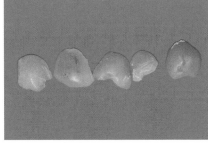

Fig 4-40 Block-out composite removed immediately after the impression is taken.

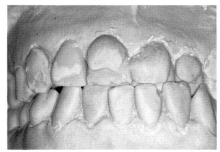

Fig 4-41 Plaster cast showing reservoirs in position prior to making the tray.

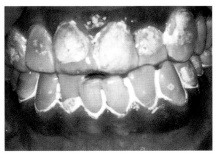

Fig 4-42 Trays in position showing reservoirs for gel.

Given the stability of tetracycline orthophosphate it might be expected that higher concentrations of carbamide peroxide might speed up bleaching. The higher the concentration of carbamide peroxide the more rapid the change in

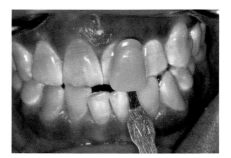

Fig 4-43 Discolouration prior to bleaching with shade tab as reference.

Fig 4-44 Results following three months of nightguard vital bleaching with 10% carbamide peroxide.

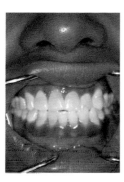

Fig 4-45 Results following six months of nightguard vital bleaching.

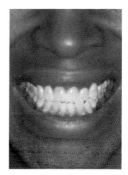

the discolouration but the greater the risk of sensitivity of the teeth. As patient compliance is a major factor with long-term bleaching, the concentration of carbamide peroxide that produces the least tooth sensitivity is the one to be preferred even though such a concentration does not result in the most rapid bleaching. The concentration of choice is 10% carbamide peroxide.

Time and Cost Implications

It takes a long time to bleach teeth affected with tetracycline orthophosphate discolouration. Tetracycline compounds are very stable, in particular in the blue/grey shade range. These compounds are much more difficult to bleach than the yellow/brown compounds. Tetracycline is only found in dentine and as a consequence the bleaching ions must penetrate deep into the tooth to have any effect.

To remember the relative difficulty of bleaching different types of tetracycline discolouration, the following may help:

| Yellow/brown | **Will** | Bleach |
| Blue/grey | **May** | Bleach |

The most difficult areas to deal with are the discoloured cervical necks of teeth, particularly if they are blue/grey in colour. The dentine is at its thickest in this area and the enamel covering it is at its thinnest. Assuming that there are no adverse effects it is worthwhile persevering with prolonged bleaching.

Alternative treatment options typically involve substantial reduction of tooth tissue and the possibility of subsequent recession exposing crown or veneer margins with three-colour transitions – white porcelain, a dark root and receded pink gingival tissues.

Different tetracycline discolourations bleach at different rates. The yellow/light brown discolourations caused by oxytetracycline bleach relatively quickly while the very dark and blue/grey discolourations are very slow to bleach. Even with protracted bleaching over many months the improvement achieved may not meet patients' reasonable expectations.

There is some evidence that patients who persevere with prolonged bleaching tend to accept the "best possible" if not ideal result. It is wise to be cautious and not to promise too much improvement. It is always better to be somewhat pessimistic and over-deliver than to raise hopes and under-deliver.

Given the length of the bleaching process necessary to manage tetracycline discolouration it is prudent not to specify the anticipated time necessary to complete treatment but to indicate that the outcome and the time taken will be largely dependent on patient compliance. This subtle transfer of responsibility back to the patient and away from the clinician is very important, in particular when prolonged bleaching is required.

The cost of supplying the large amount of gel required needs to be considered. If the diagnosis is tetracycline discolouration then arrangements can be made for the patient to receive at least a three-month supply of gel, possibly in three batches, each sufficient to last a month. The patient should be advised to keep the gel in a cool place. Given the safety of prolonged bleaching, the first recall can be at three months unless the patient suffers any adverse effects or if bleaching occurs quicker than anticipated.

Further supplies of gel can then be issued, as required. It is sensible to keep contemporaneous written records of the gel provided, together with a record of the repeated warnings being given about patient compliance being the key to success.

Congenital Conditions

Dentinogenesis Imperfecta

Dentinogenesis imperfecta is a localised form of mesodermal dysplasia of the dentine. It affects both the primary and permanent dentitions. Dentinogenesis imperfecta is the most common dental genetic disorder and affects about one in 8000 live births. It is an autosomal dominant condition with variable expressivity. It is equally distributed between sexes but predominantly seen in white people.

Primary teeth are normally more severely affected than permanent teeth. In Type I, dentine mineralisation defects are coupled with osteogenesis imperfecta. In Type II, often referred to as "hereditary opalescent dentine", which affects the permanent dentition, the dentinal defects are not related to any other collagen defects. The Type III "brandy wine" type is very rare.

Clinical appearance
Teeth affected by dentinogenesis imperfecta vary in colour from yellow/brown to brownish violet/grey with atypical translucency and opalescence (Figs 4-46 and 4-47).

The atypical colour of the teeth is caused by dentine showing through the relatively translucent opalescent enamel. Because of the abnormal scalloping along the dentine–enamel junction, the enamel tends to chip and fracture off the tips of the teeth. Loss of the enamel leads to the dentine being exposed thereby leaving the occlusal surfaces of the posterior teeth flat.

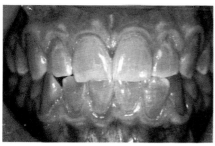

Fig 4-46 Dentinogenesis imperfecta.

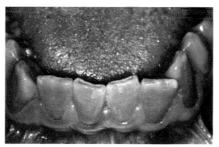

Fig 4-47 Dentinogenesis imperfecta – lower arch.

71

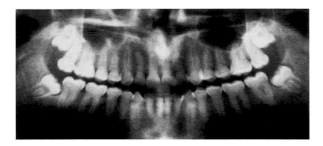

Fig 4-48 Radiographic appearance of dentinogenesis imperfecta.

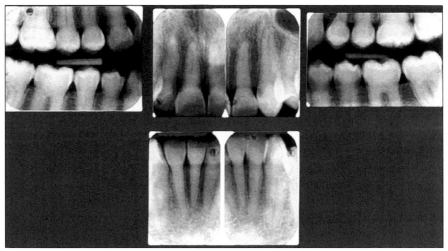

Fig 4-49 Radiographic appearance. Note the absence of pulp chambers and root canals.

The pulp canals are progressively obliterated through continuing formation of dentine. The roots are often short and blunt. The periodontal membranes and supporting bone appear normal (Figs 4-48 and 4-49).

Treatment
The aim of treatment in the management of dentinogenesis imperfecta is to provide the patient with a reasonable appearance at an early age, to maintain the occlusal vertical dimension by limiting attrition and to avoid any interference with the eruption of the other permanent teeth.

Many restorative options have been proposed. These include: overlay dentures, stainless steel crowns (with or without facings), simple removable appliances, adhesive restorations, and cast metal ceramic restorations.

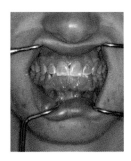

Fig 4-50
Dentino-
genesis
imperfecta
before
bleaching.

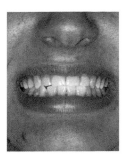

Fig 4-51
Results after
bleaching.

Following bleaching, roughened areas can be covered with conventional resin-bonded composite. This bonding should be delayed following bleaching for at least one week to preclude the possibility of any weakening of the composite bond.

Adhesive metal castings and direct composite restorations do not cause long-term biological problems. Aggressive prosthodontic therapy and removable prostheses may over time further compromise the dental status of the patient. Bleaching, notably prolonged nightguard vital bleaching, can greatly improve the treatment outcome. Chair-side bleaching tends to be ineffective. Strips impregnated with hydrogen peroxide are unlikely to be helpful given the need for repeated, prolonged bleaching to achieve any real effect.

Little attention has been paid to the psychological benefits of bleaching in patients affected by dentinogenesis imperfecta. Bleaching removes one of the main reasons for social isolation in young people with the condition. In the case illustrated in Figs 4-50 and 4-51 nightguard vital bleaching was undertaken over a period of eight months. There was a very gradual change in colour but this was sufficient to give the patient new confidence and a willingness to socialise.

The risk of sensitivity during prolonged bleaching in patients with dentinogenesis imperfecta is very low given the obliteration of the pulps by the continuous dentine deposition. In the case illustrated, the patient reported no sensitivity. The standard method of blocking out the cast to create reservoirs before making the tray was employed. A total of 142 tubes of 10% carbamide peroxide were used without any adverse side-effects. The cost of the minimally invasive approach offered by bleaching was a fraction of the estimated cost of more aggressive approaches to the management of the problem.

The psychological effects of bleaching had a profound effect on this patient's social interaction. Initially he was very shy, did not smile and put his hand over his mouth during normal conversation. At about four months he had gained some confidence and at eight months he laughed openly without trying to hide his teeth with his hand.

Amelogenesis Imperfecta

Amelogenesis imperfecta is transmitted as an autosomal-dominant sex-linked recessive trait or as a sex-linked dominant trait (Figs 4-52 to 4-57). It can be manifested as hypoplasia, hypomaturation or hypocalcification.

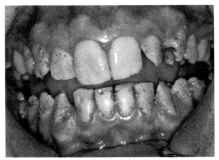

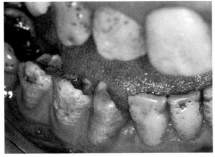

Fig 4-52 Amelogenesis imperfecta before bleaching. Note the missing upper left canine and the rotated upper left first premolar.

Fig 4-53 Amelogenesis imperfecta – rough hypoplastic type. Note the rotated lower right canine.

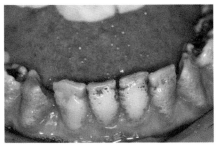

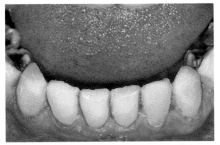

Fig 4-54 Close-up of lower teeth.

Fig 4-55 Following bleaching and direct composite application. No enamel was removed.

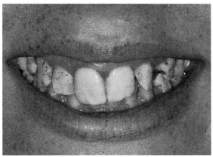

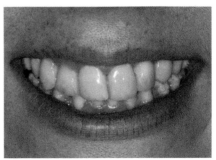

Fig 4-56 Labial view prior to bleaching.

Fig 4-57 After bleaching and bonding with direct composite.

Hypoplasia, hypocalcification, hypomaturation
Enamel hypoplasia can occur in the first stages of enamel matrix formation or during the second stage when most of the matrix is calcified. Systemic and local factors can affect normal formation of the enamel matrix causing enamel hypoplasia. If calcification is disrupted the result is enamel hypocalcification.

Hypoplasia can be mild or severe with marked pitting or irregular banding of the crowns of the teeth. Hypoplasia in the primary teeth is not normally as severe as that seen in the permanent dentition.

Hypoplastic and hypocalcified enamel are readily stained and abraded. Hypomaturation results in thin, smooth hypoplastic enamel that is relatively susceptible to abrasion and caries.

Further Reading

Aldred MJ, Savarirayan R, Crawford PJ. Amelogenesis imperfecta: a classification and catalogue for the 21st century. Oral Dis 2003;9:19–23.

Aoba T, Fejerskov O. Dental fluorosis; chemistry and biology. Crit Rev Oral Biol Med 2002;13:155–170.

Ayaslioglu E, Erkek E, Oba AA. Doxycylcine-induced staining of permanent adult dentition. Aust Dent J 2005;50:273–275.

Davies AK, Cundall RB, Dandiker Y, Slifkin MA. Photo oxidation of tetracycline absorbed on hydroxyapatite in relation to the light-induced staining of teeth. J Dent Res 1985;64:936–939.

Evelander G, Rolle GK, Cohlan SQ. The effect of the administration of tetracycline on the development of teeth. J Dent Res 1961;40:220–224.

Levy SM. An update on fluoride and fluorosis. J Can Dent Assoc 2003;69: 286–291.

Thylstrup A, Fejerskov O. Clinical appearance of dental fluorosis in permanent teeth in relation to histologic changes. Community Dent Oral Epidemiol 1978; 6:315–328.

Warren JJ, Levy SM. A review of dentifrice related to dental fluorosis. Pediatr Dent 1999;21:265–271.

Witkop CJ. Amelogenesis imperfecta, dentinogenesis imperfecta and dentin dysplasia revisited: problems in classification. J Oral Pathol 1988;17:547–553.

Chapter 5
Chair-side Bleaching

Aim

To give an overview of chair-side bleaching and to evaluate the contribution of heat and light to accelerating the process.

Outcome

The practitioner will be more informed about the controversies surrounding chair-side bleaching, particularly in relation to claims made for the efficacy of customised lights on bleaching.

Chair-side Bleaching

Chair-side bleaching is also known as *power bleaching* or *in-surgery bleaching*.

History

The first use of hydrogen peroxide for dental bleaching is attributed to Harlan in 1884. He called hydrogen peroxide "hydrogen dioxide". Its use was said to be applicable in the management of all discolourations of teeth. In 1910, Prinz described the use of 30% hydrogen peroxide on live and dead teeth. In 1918, Abbot reported that high-intensity light accelerated tooth bleaching with hydrogen peroxide. In 1924, Prinz described the use of a mixture of perborate and hydrogen peroxide, activated by a light source in order to accelerate bleaching.

To increase the effectiveness of chair-side bleaching, heat was used to help speed up the rate of disassociation of a highly concentrated preparation of hydrogen peroxide. This approach was deemed necessary to save clinical time. Chair-side time was, and remains, a valuable commodity, but as the high-concentration chemicals necessary are caustic and damaging to soft tissues, the advantages of the time saved must be weighed against the risks and nature of the possible adverse side-effects.

Mechanism

The consecutive conjugated double bonds within the discolouring molecules need to be broken down by the hydrogen peroxide. For this to happen, hydrogen peroxide has to release perhydroxyl ions continuously while the material is kept in contact with the teeth but away from the soft tissues.

Technique

Patient Assessment

All dental procedures have advantages and disadvantages. Assessment of patient expectations of bleaching is extremely important and should be done at the earliest opportunity. Patient management is discussed in detail in Chapter 2.

Safety

Gloves, masks and eye protection are essential for all team members throughout the chair-side bleaching procedure. Full protection should also be used when cleaning up. Patients must wear protective glasses. They should be advised in advance that they will not be able to touch their face during the procedure and they should keep their hands underneath the non-absorbent protective bib throughout.

Prophylaxis with a slurry of pumice and water, possibly following ultrasonic cleaning of the teeth, is indicated prior to bleaching in order to remove extrinsic stains, other deposits and salivary pellicle. It is important that teeth are cleaned thoroughly prior to the application of the rubber dam.

Isolation of the Teeth

Great care needs to be taken to ensure that the soft tissues remain protected throughout the bleaching procedure when applying high-concentration hydrogen peroxide gel. Teeth to be bleached must be fully included in the rubber dam, with the dam inverted into the gingival sulcus to ensure bleaching of the necks of the teeth. Rubber dam is not an optional extra. When high-concentration hydrogen peroxide comes in contact with soft tissue there is profound blanching followed by a marked inflammatory response. Prolonged contact, as may occur where the rubber dam does not fully protect the underlying soft tissue, may result in epithelial sloughing and ulceration. This may result in localised recession on healing, or possibly the loss of one or more interdental papillae, altering the gingival contour and significantly compromising the aesthetic outcome of the treatment.

Painful burns to the skin have been the source of litigation in the past. Damage to patients' eyes through accidental splashing of the hydrogen peroxide preparation is the most serious possible consequence.

Isolation using rubber dam and caulking material
It is important to punch and fit the rubber dam carefully around the necks of the teeth. In practical terms, the difficult areas to isolate are the cervical margins. In addition, it is prudent to use a separate caulking system (Oraseal, Ultradent Products Inc.) underneath the dam to give extra protection to the soft tissues. If the necks of the teeth are to be bleached, then the dam needs to be inverted. Any caulking material that may have escaped on to the teeth from below the dam needs to be removed before the bleaching gel is applied (see Figs 5-1 to 5-3). Fig 5-4 shows sclerosed teeth prior to bleaching.

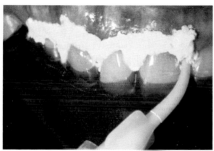

Fig 5-1 Caulking system in place. (Figure courtesy of Dan Fischer, Ultradent Products Inc.)

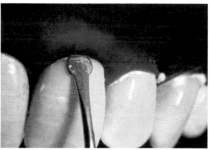

Fig 5-2 Rubber dam inverted. (Figure courtesy of Dan Fischer, Ultradent Products Inc.)

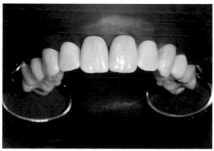

Fig 5-3 Rubber dam in position. (Figure courtesy of Dan Fischer, Ultradent Products Inc.)

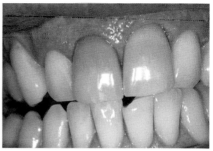

Fig 5-4 Sclerosed teeth prior to bleaching.

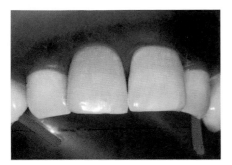

Fig 5-5 Rubber dam with Wedjets (Hygenic Corp., Akron) and prior to floss ligatures being placed.

Wedjets (Hygenic Corp., Akron) can help to secure the rubber dam in difficult situations (Fig 5-5).

Using rubber dam and floss
Floss ligatures can be tied around the necks of the teeth to help keep the rubber dam in position. The ligatures must be made of waxed dental floss (see Figs 5-6 and 5-7). Unwaxed dental floss will act as a wick to draw up the hydrogen peroxide gel by capillary action. This may result in burns to the gingival tissues.

Plastic rather than metal rubber dam clamps will prevent a build-up of heat. An absorbent tissue is placed over the lower face to protect the lower lip and chin from any gel that may be accidentally splashed or dropped during the procedure.

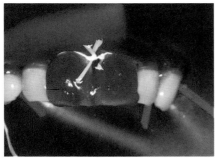

Fig 5-6 Waxed dental floss in position.

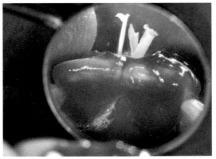

Fig 5-7 Palatal view of 38% hydrogen peroxide gel in position. Note floss ligatures and bubbling.

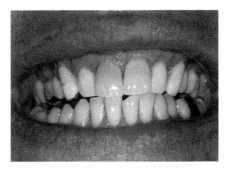

Fig 5-8 Teeth one week after chair-side bleaching – only modest improvement.

It should be noted that the placement of rubber dam and inversion of the dam into the gingival crevices is not pleasant and sometimes can be painful for patients.

Fig 5-8 shows the teeth one week following chair-side bleaching. If bleaching teeth following orthodontic treatment, it is important to "check etch" the teeth to verify that the orthodontic resin cement has been removed. If resin tags are still present in the enamel, the areas formerly covered by the bracket cement will become apparent following etching. This residual composite needs to be cut back with a multibladed plain-cut tungsten carbide bur (Jet FG 7901) in a high-speed handpiece, with a light touch to minimise enamel damage, and a dry field to see the composite more clearly. The removal of the resin-impregnated enamel to a depth of 50 microns is all that is required to allow uniform bleaching of the tooth surface.

Etching of the teeth with ortho-phosphoric acid has been suggested to enhance the penetration of hydrogen peroxide. In general terms, such etching, or indeed any etching, is neither essential nor beneficial to the clinical outcome of bleaching.

Sensitivity

Severe pain has been reported with chair-side bleaching, usually within 24 hours. This pain is caused by reversible pulpitis. Patients need to be aware of the risk of severe sensitivity before giving consent to the use of high-concentration hydrogen peroxide. If teeth are sensitive following chair-side bleaching, the wearing of a customised mouthguard with a gel or toothpaste containing 5% potassium nitrate can be helpful in controlling the symptoms.

The Bleaching Material

The bleaching material of choice is a thick gel that can be easily applied and placed accurately, without it running off the teeth. One delivery system involves mixing together the contents of two tubes by interlocking them (38% hydrogen peroxide, Ultradent Products Inc.) and pressing the material from one tube to the other until the 38% hydrogen peroxide gel is fully mixed. The gel is red, enabling the operator to see where the material is being placed (Fig 5-9). Once mixed, the gel must be used relatively quickly, typically within 10 days.

Storage
High concentration bleaching gels are unstable with variations in temperature so care has to be taken to keep them refrigerated. This is critical to the shelf-life of the material.

Application of Bleaching Material
The bleaching gel, which usually contains between 15% and 38% hydrogen peroxide, is applied to all the teeth to be bleached at the same time and left in position for about 15 minutes. The gel should be agitated. Light or heat can be used in an attempt to speed up the process (Fig 5-10) but the benefit of this is questionable.

The gel is washed off every 15 minutes, the teeth are dried and new bleaching material is applied. High-volume aspiration is the most convenient way of removing the bulk of the gel. This should be done *before* any residual material

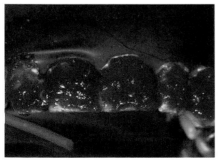

Fig 5-9 The 38% hydrogen peroxide bleaching gel in place.

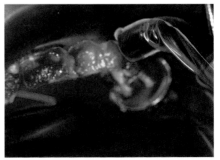

Fig 5-10 Light being used on the bleaching gel.

is washed off. This will ensure there is a minimal amount of gel remaining to be washed away using the three-in-one syringe. Adhering to this procedure will limit the risks of splashing.

This procedure needs to be repeated three to four times. It is therefore prudent to allow about 90 minutes of chair-side time for this. A lot of this clinical time is taken up placing the rubber dam, applying the caulking paste, and otherwise taking precautions to ensure that the gel does not come into contact with soft tissue, in particular the gingivae. During the bleaching procedure, the patient must be supervised and assisted, if necessary, with the removal of excess saliva from under the rubber dam. All in all, this is a procedure which is costly in terms of dental team chair-side time.

Acceleration Techniques

Acceleration of chair-side bleaching can be attempted in various ways.

Increasing the Concentration of Hydrogen Peroxide

The higher the concentration of hydrogen peroxide the quicker the oxidation process will proceed. In this context, a high concentration usually means 25–38% hydrogen peroxide. Manufacturers normally state the effective concentration of hydrogen peroxide in the gel but some information leaflets can be confusing, if not actually misleading, in this regard. Knowing the concentration of the material selected is critical to understanding the inherent risks in using the gel and to taking appropriate measures to protect the patient and members of the dental team.

Use of Light-activated Catalysts

A light-activated catalyst may be included in the gel to allow control over the activation of the bleaching process. When the material is in position the light is used to initiate the catalytic reaction.

Use of Heat and Light

Heating the gel will increase the speed of disassociation of the hydrogen peroxide gel, making more perhydroxyl ions available for breaking down the discolouring molecules in the teeth. An increase of 10 °C doubles the rate of disassociation of hydrogen peroxide. If the application of heat is used to increase the rate of bleaching, it is necessary to increase the temperature *inside* the substance of the teeth, where the discolouring molecules are present. An increase in the temperature of the gel on the surface of the teeth alone will have little, if any, effect.

It is important when applying heat that the teeth are not anaesthetised so the patients can report any discomfort caused by the increase in temperature. Generally speaking, if patients do not report discomfort when the material is being heated, it means that the pulps of the teeth are unlikely to be damaged by the bleaching procedure.

Concentration and Efficacy

The immediate lightening effect of chair-side bleaching is related, in part, to the dehydration of the teeth being isolated under rubber dam. A high-concentration hydrogen peroxide gel bleaches more quickly than one of a low concentration. The use of high-concentration bleaching gel under rubber dam may result in an accentuated dehydration effect with a consequent "rebound" in the colour, producing a darkening of the teeth as they rehydrate.

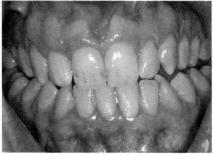

Fig 5-11 Teeth prior to chair-side bleaching.

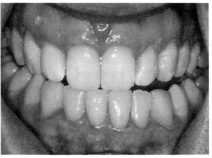

Fig 5-12 Two weeks after chair-side bleaching.

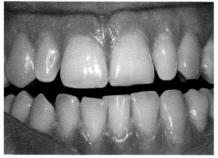

Fig 5-13 Underexposed photograph of teeth before bleaching.

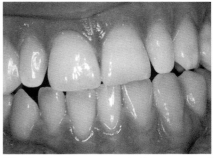

Fig 5-14 Overexposed photograph of teeth following bleaching. At least some of the effect is photographic and not clinically relevant.

It is unclear to what extent the heating of high-concentration hydrogen peroxide gels on the surface of the teeth speeds or otherwise influences these effects. Caution must be exercised in interpreting manufacturers' claims of up to eight shade-tab changes with chair-side bleaching (Figs 5-11 and 5-12).

Advertising literature can be misleading. Photographs deliberately taken with different light exposures can give the temporary illusion of dramatic tooth whitening (Figs 5-13 and 5-14).

Some clinical photographs included in advertising material would appear to have been taken immediately after the rubber dam has been removed and while the teeth were still dehydrated, thereby maximising the visual, temporary effect of the bleaching.

Manufacturers' claims for dramatic effects with chair-side systems have not been substantiated by the American Dental Association (ADA) Seal of Approval Scheme. The ADA requires that, for their approval, 85% of colour change is maintained at three months and 75% at six months. To date, none of the chair-side bleaching systems have been awarded the ADA seal of approval.

Effectiveness

Surface coatings and deposits giving rise to discolouration are lightened, but not removed, by bleaching. Superficial stains caused by tobacco, coffee or other highly coloured substances are easy to bleach but may be better managed by thorough scaling and polishing and appropriate oral hygiene instructions.

Discolouration caused by more complex molecules, in particular those including benzene rings and metal ions with consecutive conjugated double bonds within teeth, may be managed most effectively by nightguard vital bleaching but these molecules take a long time to break down and lighten. Chair-side bleaching may produce disappointing results in such cases.

Up to three or four visits may be required to complete chair-side bleaching to produce results similar to those obtainable with nightguard vital bleaching. Patients need to be aware of the time and costs involved prior to giving consent for such treatment.

One has to question, given the proven efficacy of nightguard vital bleaching, whether chair-side bleaching is a sensible use of clinical time, other than for those patients who wish and are prepared to pay for an "instant result". It is acknowledged, however, that some dentists prefer to have direct control over the bleaching processes, even if chair-side bleaching involves considerable chair-side time and may not be as effective or long-lasting as nightguard vital bleaching.

Chair-side bleaching is, however, useful for a patient with a severe gag reflex who is unable to tolerate wearing a tray for the time required to complete the bleaching.

Guarantees should not be given that chair-side bleaching will be successful. If the dentist is unsure of the cause of the discolouration (e.g. tetracycline), chair-side bleaching may be relatively costly and very ineffective in such a case. In contrast, nightguard vital bleaching may be effective in such situations but may well take between four and six months to achieve an acceptable clinical outcome (see Chapter 2).

With chair-side bleaching, the onus is on the dentist to achieve the desired bleaching outcome. In contrast, with nightguard vital bleaching the onus is on the patient.

Light-assisted Chair-side Bleaching

Controversy still exists as to the role of a light in bleaching, other than as a method of heating the material or activating a light-activated catalyst. In contrast to the evidence available in respect of nightguard vital bleaching, there is a dearth of robust evidence in respect of bleaching materials used with plasma arc or other types of light or lasers.

The use of a light or laser increases the surface temperature of the gel and initiates any light-activated catalyst within the gel. If there is no light-activated catalyst within the gel then simply heating highly concentrated hydrogen peroxide gel should speed up the rate of disassociation. If this rise in temperature were deemed to be desirable, the same effect could be achieved without a light by using simpler means such as an endodontic heating instrument commonly used for obturation.

Figs 5-15 and 5-16 show teeth before and after light-assisted chair-side bleaching.

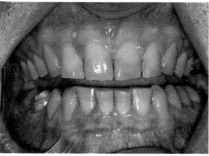
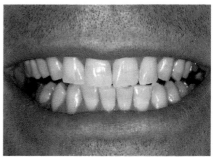

Fig 5-15 Teeth before light-assisted chair-side bleaching.

Fig 5-16 Teeth after light-assisted chair-side bleaching.

Lights and Heating Devices

Various devices have been developed for the purposes of providing heat and light which claim to accelerate the rate of bleaching. These include:
• Xenon halogen
• LED light
• Diode lasers
• Plasma Arc lamps
• Composite photoactivation units.

To date, none of the light bleaching systems have ADA approval.

Proprietary Bleaching Systems

The Illuminator (Union Broach) includes a light and a heating instrument to increase the temperature on selected parts of the teeth being bleached. The application of heat and light can be controlled separately, with gel being applied and topped up with a bleaching wand. Feedback from the patient is important in ensuring that the pulps of the teeth being bleached are not suffering any harm.

The Luma Arch system (Luma Lite Inc.) uses 35% hydrogen peroxide material with a pH of 5.5. The directions for use state that three applications of eight minutes are required together with the use of the Luma Arch light. The Luma Arch hydrogen peroxide gel is hand-mixed prior to application. The Zoom system (Discus Dental Inc.) uses 25% hydrogen peroxide with a pH of 8 along with their light. The manufacturer recommends three 20-minute applications of gel along with the use of the light in each session.

Opalescence Extra Boost uses a 38% hydrogen peroxide gel with a pH of 7. This material includes a catalyst pH adjuster, which is activated by mixing the contents of two syringes. At the preparation stage these are locked together to allow the material to be pushed back and forth to mix them. The directions for use state that the gel should be applied for 15 minutes and then replaced. Four applications are suggested in a session, with a total bleaching time of 60 minutes. A light can be used during bleaching but the manufacturer questions whether this is of any benefit.

The bleaching results achieved by using the Luma Arch, Zoom or Opalescence Extra Boost systems have been found to be similar one week after bleaching. All three systems produced 1.7 units of colour change.

Cost of Lights and Materials

Opalescence Extra Boost (38% hydrogen peroxide with catalyst) can be used with a light but it does not require one.

The Luma Arch system requires about one-third the time required for Opalescence Extra Boost – 24 minutes versus 60 minutes – but the light, which includes four xenon-halogen lamps, is expensive to purchase. The Luma Arch 35% hydrogen peroxide gel decomposes relatively rapidly with or without exposure to light by action of its chemical catalyst. This bleaching material is marginally cheaper than other high-concentration hydrogen peroxide gels.

The Zoom light, which has one high-intensity metal-halide lamp, is approximately one-third of the cost of the Luma Arch light. The Zoom material is five times more expensive than the Opalescence Extra Boost gel but includes resin for soft tissue protection, take-home bleach, bleaching tray material and a case, sun block creams and fluoride gel. The home bleach component of the system has a similar effect to standard nightguard vital bleaching. Much of the longer-term benefits claimed for bleaching with the Zoom system are probably as attributable to the home bleaching element as to the actual chair-side procedures.

Many dentists "back both horses" in that they use chair-side bleaching to kick-start tooth lightening followed by nightguard vital bleaching. The results are no better, although quicker, than with nightguard vital bleaching alone. Given the time involved in chair-side bleaching, the fees for nightguard vital bleaching alone should be more affordable and better value for the typical patient.

None of the chair-side bleaching systems are more effective than nightguard vital bleaching. Chair-side bleaching has greater equivalent costs, in particular if a proprietary light is purchased, requires more clinical time, involves higher material costs and has a much higher risk profile. The main justification for the use of chair-side bleaching is the immediate result for patients who are not prepared to tolerate or lack the patience to undertake nightguard vital bleaching.

Some papers' claims for light-augmented tooth whitening with 15% hydrogen peroxide gel used in conjunction with a plasma light have caused considerable controversy and correspondence about the dubious methods and results involved.

Bleaching lights are expensive, occupy valuable surgery space and have an unproven effect on the outcome of bleaching.

To date, none of the systems utilising "powerful" chair-side lights for bleaching have been granted ADA approval. Nightguard vital bleaching using 10% carbamide peroxide within a customised bleaching tray remains the gold standard in dental bleaching.

Further Reading

DeSilva Gottardi M, Brackett MG, Haywood VB. Number of in-office light-activated bleaching treatments needed to achieve patient satisfaction. Quintessence Int 2006;37:115–120.

Hein DK, Ploeqer BJ, Hartup JK, Wagstaff RS, Palmer TM, Hansen LD. In-office vital tooth bleaching – what do lights add? Compend Contin Educ Dent 2003;24:340–352.

Kugel G, Papathanasiou A, Williams AJ et al. Clinical evaluation of chemical and light-activated tooth whitening systems. Compend Contin Educ Dent 2006;27:54–62.

Papathanasiou A, Kastali S, Perry RD, Kugel G. Clinical evaluation of a 35% hydrogen peroxide in-office whitening system. Compend Contin Educ Dent 2002;23:335–338:340:343–344.

Sulieman M, Addy M, Macdonald E, Rees JS. A safety study in vitro for the effects of an in-office bleaching system on the integrity of enamel and dentine. J Dent 2004;32:581–590.

Swift EJ, Heymann HO, Kugel G, Kanca J. More about tooth whitening. JADA 2003;134:814–815. (This should be read in conjunction with Tavares M et al. – see below.)

Tavares M, Stultz J, Newman M, Smith V, Kent R, Carpino E, Goodson JM. Light augments tooth whitening with peroxide. J Am Dent Assoc 2003;134:167–175.

Chapter 6
Over-the-counter Bleaching Products

Aim

The aim is to familiarise practitioners with the range and use of over-the-counter (OTC) products and the problems associated with this approach to bleaching.

Outcome

Practitioners will be more familiar with the appearance issues surrounding the use of unsupervised over-the-counter products.

Introduction

Unsupervised bleaching can be cost-effective for some patients but has certain limitations and drawbacks. Restorations can appear mismatched in shade following such bleaching.

Bleaching Strips

The use of intraoral strips to deliver therapeutic agents or other substances is not new. In the past, strips have been used to deliver, for example, topical steroids in the management of conditions such as aphthous ulceration. In the past five years, a number of over-the-counter bleaching systems have been developed. These are supplied by a pharmacy or simply purchased in a supermarket without any input or prescription from a dentist.

Bleaching strips are of varying thickness and are available with different concentrations and amounts of bleaching agents. Pre-packaged products are available for maxillary and mandibular teeth. They are available in a variety of shapes, sizes and packaging, usually designed to entice consumers into the popular and lucrative market of tooth bleaching. The sale of over-the-counter bleaching systems represents huge business worldwide. Figs 6-1 to 6-4 give an example of bleaching strips available over-the-counter.

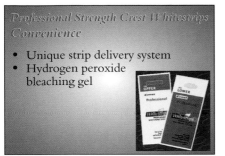

Professional Strength Crest Whitestrips
Convenience

- Unique strip delivery system
- Hydrogen peroxide bleaching gel

Fig 6-1 Professional Crest Whitestrips (Procter and Gamble).

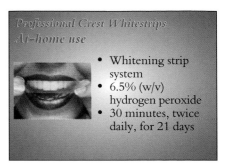

Professional Crest Whitestrips
At-home use

- Whitening strip system
- 6.5% (w/v) hydrogen peroxide
- 30 minutes, twice daily, for 21 days

Fig 6-2 Hydrogen peroxide content of strips.

Professional Crest Whitestrips
Features

- Flexible device: polyethylene strip
- Established chemistry: 6.5% (w/v) H_2O_2
- Bleaching gel: glycerin/Carbopol/water
- Low overall dose: 10-13 mg H_2O_2
- Short contact time: 30 minutes twice daily

Fig 6-3 Features of strips.

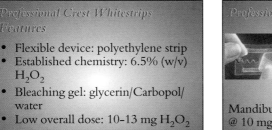

Professional Crest Whitestrips

Maxillary strip @ 13 mg hydrogen peroxide

Mandibular strip @ 10 mg hydrogen peroxide

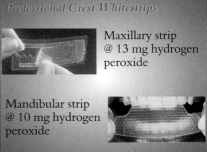

Fig 6-4 Bleaching strips contain 5–16% hydrogen peroxide.

Randomised, controlled clinical trials have shown that bleaching strips containing 10% hydrogen peroxide (equivalent to 30% carbamide peroxide) are effective if used twice daily for seven days. Fig 6-5 shows a strip in position.

Bleaching strips are generally safe. They are designed to bleach all the teeth covered by the strips. Selective bleaching of specific teeth is not possible with these products.

The thin flexible strips occupy much less space than trays used for nightguard vital bleaching but they lack the fit of customised trays. Because of the relatively poor adaptation of the strip to the underlying teeth, saliva can inactivate the hydrogen peroxide relatively easily thereby limiting the

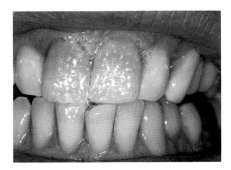

Fig 6-5 Bleaching strip in position.

effectiveness of the strip to 30 minutes and making reuse ineffective. For this reason a relatively high concentration of hydrogen peroxide is essential for the bleaching strips to be effective. Bleaching strips can be a useful alternative in the treatment of patients who have difficulty wearing a conventional nightguard bleaching tray.

Paint-on Gel

An alternative over-the-counter approach to the use of bleaching strips involves the use of a paint-on gel applied by the patient. The product contains 18% carbamide peroxide which releases the equivalent of about 6% hydrogen peroxide. The gel is designed to be painted directly on to the labial aspects of the target teeth. The findings of clinical trials of this product when directly compared to nightguard vital bleaching have not been particularly convincing.

Problems with Over-the-counter Products

The drive for over-the-counter products comes, amongst other factors, from people unwilling to consult dentists or unable to afford dentist-delivered bleaching. As with other over-the-counter therapies there is a risk that consumers fail to understand the true nature of the problem they seek to treat. In so doing they may do themselves more aesthetic harm than good in using these products.

People using over-the-counter bleaching products often fail to understand that existing restorations may not match the colour of the adjacent tooth tissue after bleaching. The use of such products can be at least disappointing and possibly very costly if subsequent restorative treatment is necessary to achieve an acceptable aesthetic result. Restorations that were a reasonable match before over-the-counter bleaching may look significantly worse after bleaching.

Matching new restorations to very bleached, almost translucent teeth can be a challenge. This can be especially difficult if the replacement restoration has a metal substructure. The hidden costs of replacing intracoronal restorations such as composites may not be excessive but the costs of extracoronal restorations, for example veneers or implant-retained crowns, may be many times greater than any saving gained by buying such over-the-counter products.

There is a strong case for all bleaching being supervised, if not actually pre-scribed, by a dentist. However, the over-the-counter market is well established and expanding largely independent of any supervision by dentists. Practitioners should be alert to the possibility that patients presenting with colour mismatched restorations may have been using over-the-counter bleaching products. Patients enquiring about bleaching should be made aware of the significant difficulties with over-the-counter products when they have existing restorations in visible anterior teeth.

Whitening Toothpastes

Claims that commercial toothpastes can lighten teeth have been made since at least the latter part of the 1880s. However, no toothpaste has been shown to produce internal lightening of teeth. Toothpastes remove extrinsic stains by means of abrasion and polishing agents. Surfactants in toothpaste help remove and prevent stain accumulation. Consequently, the effects of whitening toothpastes tend to be superficial and transient.

Within the European Community the amount of hydrogen peroxide permitted in toothpaste is limited to 0.1%. At this level, whitening toothpastes are hopelessly ineffective as bleaching agents. Any hydrogen peroxide released from the toothpaste will be rapidly inactivated by saliva.

Consumers can be confused by unsubstantiated claims and packaging. This confusion is further compounded by some manufacturers producing toothpastes with the same name as their 10% carbamide peroxide products which are designed for nightguard vital bleaching.

Further Reading

Brunton PA, Aminian A, Pretty IA. Vital tooth bleaching in dental practice: 2. Novel bleaching systems. Dent Update 2006;33:357–358:360–362.

Gerlach RW, Sagel PA, Barker ML et al. Vital bleaching with a thin peroxide gel: the safety and efficacy of a professional strength hydrogen peroxide whitening strip. J Am Dent Assoc 2004;135:98–100.

Kapinia K, Magnusson I, Barker ML, Gerlach RW. Clinical comparison of two self directed bleaching systems. J Prosthodont 2003;12:242–248.

Shahidi H, Barker ML, Sagel PA, Gerlach RW. Randomized control trials of 10% hydrogen peroxide whitening strips. J Clin Dent 2005;16:91–95.

Zantner C, Derdilopoulou M, Martus P et al. Randomized clinical trial on the efficacy of two over-the-counter whitening systems. Quintessence Int 2006; 37:695–706.

Chapter 7

Frequently Asked Questions

Aim

This chapter asks and answers the most frequently asked questions.

Outcome

Practitioners will be able to answer the most common queries that patients have about bleaching.

What Causes Tooth Discolouration?

Tooth discolouration is caused by external (extrinsic) or internal (intrinsic) colourants or a combination of both (see Tables 7-1 and 7-2 and Figs 7-1 to 7-10).

Are There Any Other Causes of Discolouration?

There are other causes of discolouration which have more pathological origins. These are outlined in Table 7-3 (page 100) and illustrated in Figs 7-11 to 7-15.

What Happens During Bleaching?

Hydrogen peroxide penetrates through the enamel and dentine, reacting with discolouration within the tooth. Discolourations, including those on external tooth surfaces, are oxidised. Discolourations in enamel usually bleach relatively quickly while those in dentine take longer to bleach.

Are There Any Contraindications to Bleaching Teeth?

Yes. Existing fillings, veneers and crowns will not change colour. If tooth-coloured restorations match the existing teeth before bleaching, they will appear darker after the natural teeth have been bleached. This may mean that existing restorations, veneers or crowns may need to be replaced following bleaching. This may add greatly to the cost of treatment.

Table 7-1 **Extrinsic colourants**

Colour	Cause
Brown or black	Tea/coffee/iron
Yellow or brown	Poor oral hygiene/tea
Yellow/brown/black	Tobacco/marijuana
Green/orange/black/brown	Bacteria
Red/purple/brown	Red wine

Table 7-2 **Intrinsic colourants**

Colour	Cause
Grey/brown/black	Pulp with haemorrhage
Yellow/grey	Pulp necrosis without haemorrhage
Brown/grey/black	Endodontic materials within the tooth
Yellow/brown	Pulpal obliteration/sclerosis
Brown/white lines/spots	Fluorosis (excessive fluoride swallowed during tooth development)
Black	Sulphur
Brown/grey	Minocycline taken after tooth formation (adult teeth)
Yellow/brown/grey/blue	Tetracycline taken during tooth development
	Doxycycline taken after tooth formation
Pink	Internal resorption
Grey/brown/black	Dental decay
Yellow/brown	Ageing

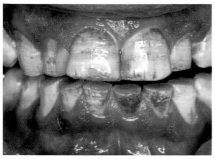

Fig 7-1 Extrinsic discolouration.

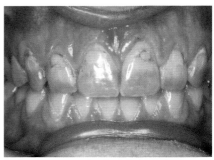

Fig 7-2 Intrinsic discolouration.

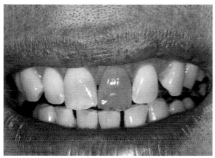

Fig 7-3 Pulp necrosis with haemorrhage.

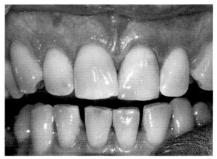

Fig 7-4 Following inside/outside bleaching and shortening.

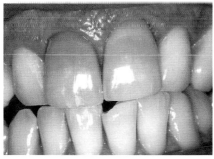

Fig 7-5 Sclerosis of both upper and central incisors.

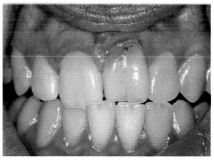

Fig 7-6 Internal and external resoption.

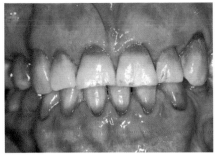

Fig 7-7 Cervical tetracycline discolouration.

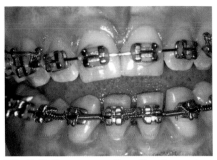

Fig 7-8 Oxytetracycline discolouration with orthodontic bands in position.

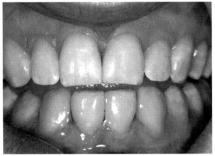

Fig 7-9 Following bleaching and direct composite bonding. (Photograph courtesy of Richard Porter).

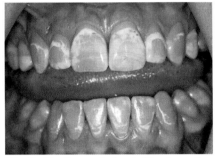

Fig 7-10 Enamel decalcification after orthodontic treatment.

Table 7-3 **Other causes of discolouration**

Colour	Cause
Yellow/brown	Amelogenesis imperfecta
Brown/violet/yellow brown	Dentinogenesis imperfecta
Brown	Inborn errors of metabolism, e.g. phenylketonurea
Black	Porphyria

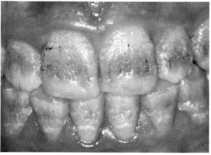

Fig 7-11 Amelogenesis imperfecta – hypoplastic type.

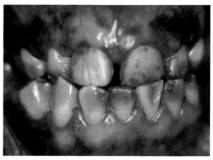

Fig 7-12 Amelogenesis imperfecta – hypomaturation.

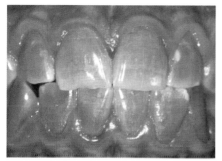

Fig 7-13 Dentinogenesis imperfecta.

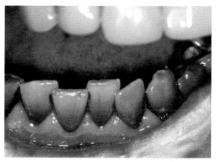

Fig 7-14 Porphyria.

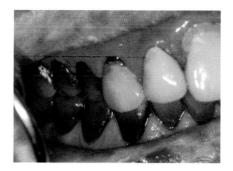

Fig 7-15 Porphyria – lower arch. Note failing crowns 10 years post-placement.

How Much will it Cost?

This varies according to the system being used, the severity of the problem, the condition of the discoloured teeth and the amount of time and material needed to achieve a satisfactory result.

Does the Patient Have to Sleep with the Bleaching Tray or Mouth-guard in Position?

Sleeping with the tray in position is the most effective way of keeping the bleaching gel in contact with the teeth for prolonged periods of time. If this is a problem, then provided the loaded tray can be worn for at least two hours each day, bleaching will be effective, but will simply take longer.

Are there any Side-effects?

The majority of patients suffer mild sensitivity during treatment. This typically resolves once bleaching has stopped. If the teeth are sensitive before bleaching, they will probably become more sensitive during bleaching.

There have been no reports of long-term side-effects of using nightguard vital bleaching with 10% carbamide peroxide. Even prolonged (six to nine months) nightguard vital bleaching has been shown to be safe (Fig 7-16).

Can the Sensitivity be Reduced?

There are a number of ways of controlling sensitivity. Desensitising tooth-pastes (usually those containing 5% potassium nitrate) can be used for two

A study of nightguard vital bleaching of tetracycline-stained teeth for six months showed that none of the patients had to have root canal treatment or had continuing sensitivity as a result of **six months** bleaching.

Leonard et al. *J Esthet Restor Dent. 2003*

Fig 7-16 Safety of long-term bleaching.

weeks prior to bleaching. Alternatively, desensitising toothpaste can be placed in the tray and worn for about half an hour before each period of bleaching. The toothpaste is then replaced with the bleaching gel. To limit the risk of sensitivity the tray with the bleaching gel may be worn for two hours only, rather than overnight.

If the teeth are sensitive prior to bleaching, the bleaching gel should not be applied more than once a day or night and the tray should be worn only for a few hours. Higher-concentration bleaching agents, for example 22% carbamide peroxide, should not be used where there is sensitivity.

Which Toothpaste Should be Used when Bleaching?

There is some evidence that brushing with a toothpaste containing 5% potassium nitrate for two weeks prior to bleaching helps reduce the risk of sensitivity. Normal toothpaste is usually used during bleaching. Toothpastes will not bleach teeth but brushing with a good-quality toothpaste can help reduce stain formation.

How Long will Bleaching Take?

This depends on the cause of the discolouration and patient compliance. It usually takes between two and six weeks of nightguard vital bleaching for normal teeth to become lighter. Tobacco discolouration takes three to six months to bleach provided the patient stops smoking. Yellow/brown tetracycline discolouration may take up to nine months to bleach. Deeply coloured blue/grey tetracycline discolouration is very difficult to bleach satisfactorily but there is usually some improvement with very prolonged bleaching.

Is Chair-side (also Known as "Power" or "In-surgery") Bleaching Better than Nightguard Vital Bleaching?

The short answer is no. There is very limited scientific evidence supporting the long-term efficacy of light-assisted chair-side bleaching. The gold standard is nightguard vital bleaching using 10% carbamide peroxide. This method has the American Dental Association (ADA) seal of approval. Light-assisted chair-side bleaching is useful for patients unable to tolerate wearing a bleaching tray and in situations in which a "kick-start" to bleaching may be advantageous.

How Long does Bleaching Last?

The effects of nightguard vital bleaching last on average two to three years before there is any noticeable deterioration. The colour change can remain stable for up to seven years, but bleached teeth may need some "top-up" bleaching at two- to three-yearly intervals. If additional bleaching is required, the time taken is normally much less than that required for the initial bleaching. As a general rule, topping up takes one night for each week taken to complete the initial bleaching.

What is the Best Material to Use?

The most extensively researched material is 10% carbamide peroxide, containing 3.5% hydrogen peroxide. The typical presentation is a thick gel for use in a customised bleaching tray made from an accurate impression of the teeth. Details of products with the ADA seal of approval are included in the Association website: www.ada.org/ada/seal/company_professional.asp.

Why Not Use Over-the-counter Products as Advertised on TV and in Magazines?

Bleaching is best managed by a dentist, who will diagnose the cause of the discolouration, assess the risk of any possible adverse effects and, where indicated, supervise bleaching, possibly as part of a more extensive treatment plan. This helps avoid colour-mismatching of teeth and restorations.

Many of the over-the-counter products have no proof of their safety or efficacy. Some products contain acids which may etch and damage the teeth and others contain titanium dioxide, as used in white paints. The titanium dioxide may whiten teeth but the effect is typically very short-lived. Many of the claims made in respect of over-the-counter products are considered to be misleading. "Boil and bite" mouthguards for use with over-the-counter bleaching gels do not fit well. As a consequence they can be uncomfortable and may fail to protect the gel from salivary deactivation, thereby producing a very disappointing result.

Are Whitening Toothpastes Effective?

Whitening toothpastes primarily remove superficial stains. Most whitening toothpastes contain only 0.1% hydrogen peroxide. None have been shown to be effective at bleaching intrinsic discolouration. A regular toothpaste used together with a proper brushing technique may be just as effective as a whitening toothpaste in removing superficial extrinsic stains.

How Much Carbamide Peroxide Gel is Swallowed During Bleaching with a Bleaching Tray?

About 25% of the carbamide peroxide gel in the tray is swallowed. Most of the hydrogen peroxide which escapes from the tray is immediately inactivated by saliva before it is swallowed. Exposure to hydrogen peroxide is at its highest when the tray is inserted. The exposure reduces rapidly over time.

Is Swallowing Hydrogen Peroxide Harmful?

Most of the hydrogen peroxide released into the mouth during bleaching is inactivated by normal saliva before being swallowed. Any gel that is swallowed is readily inactivated in the stomach. Any hydrogen peroxide that is absorbed and enters the circulation is quickly and effectively inactivated by red blood cells.

The answers to less frequently asked questions will be found in other chapters of this book.

Further Reading

Haywood VB. Frequently asked questions about bleaching. Compend Contin Educ Dent 2003;24:324–338.

Leonard RH, Haywood VB, Caplan DJ, Tart ND. Nightguard vital bleaching of tetracycline-stained teeth 90 months post treatment. J Esthet Restore Dent. 2003;15:142-152. Discussion 153.

Chapter 8

Information for Patients

Aim

This chapter provides "takeaway" information that can usefully be included in practice information leaflets.

Outcome

Practitioners will be aware of the information that patients may need in relation to bleaching. Making this information available may form part of the consent process.

Nightguard Vital Bleaching

Nightguard vital bleaching involves wearing a customised bleaching tray or mouthguard containing bleaching gel. The gel releases a low concentration of hydrogen peroxide, which bleaches discolouring stains both on the surface and within the body of teeth. The tray, which is a thin version of a protective sports mouthguard, is usually worn overnight with the gel in it. Treatment normally takes about four to six weeks but some discolouration, such as that caused by tetracycline antibiotics taken in childhood, can take many months to lighten. Nightguard vital bleaching offers a safe and effective method of bleaching moderately discoloured teeth.

What Does Nightguard Vital Bleaching Involve?

The treatment usually involves three visits to the dentist. The first visit includes an examination, a medical and dental history, and radiographs (x-rays) of the teeth being taken if necessary. The causes of any discolouration will be established by the dentist. Tests may be undertaken to determine whether the nerves of the teeth to be bleached are alive or dead. If the teeth are dead or have decay these problems need to be dealt with before bleaching.

If there are tooth-coloured restorations present the possible effects of bleaching need to be carefully considered. If bleaching is undertaken it is likely that certain restorations may need to be changed following bleaching. This will need to be discussed as well as the associated fees involved for doing this.

The gums will be examined for gum disease and the possibility of recession. Thin gums are likely to be associated with sensitivity during bleaching.

The teeth will be tested for sensitivity, probably by blowing cold air on them. If they are sensitive to start with, this sensitivity will probably increase temporarily with bleaching.

If it is decided to go ahead with bleaching, impressions and photographs will be taken. It is common practice to treat the teeth in one arch and use the other arch as a control. Patients may or may not want the teeth in both arches bleached. This should be discussed with the dentist.

If a partial denture is being worn and it is desired to bleach the teeth at night and during the day then two separate trays need to be made, from two separate impressions. One impression will be made with, and one without, the removable denture in position.

At the second visit the tray will be tried in position and adjusted as necessary. Instructions will be given on the use of the tray and the appropriate amount of bleaching gel dispensed. The gel should be kept in a cool place. Instructions will be given on how to load the tray with the bleaching gel and how to insert it. A follow-up appointment will be arranged to evaluate progress.

How Long Does it Take?
It is difficult to predict how long it will take for bleaching to be effective but the dentist will be able to give "a best guess" as to how long it is likely to take. The time taken varies between patients and may be influenced by a number of factors.

The more the gel-loaded tray is worn the quicker bleaching will occur. As an alternative to night-time wear the tray can be worn during the day except when eating and cleaning the teeth. The gel needs to be changed every six hours. If the tray cannot be worn continuously for at least two hours then bleaching is unlikely to be very successful if using 10% carbamide peroxide.

Will I Have to Keep Bleaching?
It is not advisable to repeat the bleaching of the satisfactorily bleached teeth unless there is an appreciable relapse in their colour. This is unlikely to happen for quite a few years. It is not advisable to bleach teeth to a level where they become unnaturally lightened.

It has been reported that four years after bleaching, 80% of teeth had maintained the lightening effect. It is easy to top up the bleaching effect by repeating the night-time bleaching at a rate of one night for each week of the original treatment time. In other words, if it took four weeks to lighten the teeth to the desired level it will take four nights to return the teeth to the desired colour. The tray used in the initial bleaching should be kept for any subsequent top-up bleaching.

Is it Safe?

Extensive research, including many clinical trials, has shown that dental bleaching with low concentrations of bleaching gels, such as 10% carbamide peroxide, is very safe. Bleaching has no long-term detrimental effects on either the dental hard tissues (enamel and dentine) or the soft tissues (gums, lining of the mouth) or nerves (pulps) of the teeth.

Bleaching with high concentrations of hydrogen peroxide is safe only provided it is undertaken by a dentist utilising a meticulous clinical technique as specified by the manufacturer of the bleach.

Is it Effective?

Clinical studies on bleaching report a success rate in excess of 80%, with the majority of patients experiencing at least some lightening. Not all teeth respond at the same speed or to the same extent. While the dentist will assess individual requirements, the real test is for the patient to try bleaching and see how it goes.

When Does it Work?

Discolouration linked to ageing and diet

Teeth that have darkened through ageing or have become stained, for example by drinking red wine or lots of coffee or tea, bleach very well. If the teeth do not respond relatively quickly it is usually a matter of extending the treatment time or using more gel for longer periods of time, to achieve the desired outcome.

Fluorosis

Fluorosis causes brown spots or white flecks, or banding on teeth. It is caused by exposure to too much fluoride when the teeth are developing. It is often caused by children swallowing rather than spitting out fluoride toothpaste at an early age.

Brown fluorosis responds moderately well to bleaching. White flecks, which are usually less obvious and therefore cause less concern, can become more obvious during bleaching because the teeth become "blotchy". This is not normally a problem once the bleaching has been completed as the white flecks tend to blend in with the lightened enamel. This outcome of bleaching is usually acceptable to most patients.

Tetracycline discolouration
Tetracycline discolouration is one of the types of discolouration least responsive to bleaching. This staining is caused by taking a particular antibiotic while the teeth are forming. Taking antibiotics containing tetracycline for prolonged periods, for example in the treatment of acne, can cause discolouration of fully erupted teeth.

Will There be Problems with Existing Restorations, Fillings or Crowns?
Bleaching will not change the colour of tooth-coloured materials used in fillings, veneers, crowns, bridges or dentures. As a result the restorations which previously matched the teeth may look darker following bleaching. If the mismatch in colour is a problem it may be necessary for at least some restorations to be replaced or resurfaced after bleaching. This may involve considerable cost, which needs to be discussed, understood and accepted before bleaching is undertaken.

If fillings, veneers, crowns or dentures are *lighter* than the natural teeth to be bleached it is sometimes possible to bleach the teeth to match the existing restorations.

If any restoration is *darker* than the adjacent tooth tissue then it will look significantly worse in terms of colour match after bleaching. The dentist will advise if this is likely to be a problem.

What about Side-effects?
Sensitivity
Most patients undergoing bleaching report some mild sensitivity. The best indicator of possible increased sensitivity during bleaching is sensitivity of the teeth prior to bleaching.

Sensitivity usually subsides one to two days after bleaching. If the problem persists, toothpaste containing 5% potassium nitrate can be placed in the tray and worn for about half an hour before using the bleaching gel. There is some evidence that brushing teeth with this type of toothpaste for two weeks prior to starting bleaching can reduce sensitivity. Alternatively, a variety of materials and chair-side techniques can be used by the dentist to manage sensitivity. If teeth are already sensitive, this should be drawn to the dentist's attention at the consultation stage.

If bleaching causes sensitivity, the gel should be changed only once a day/night. Higher concentrations of bleaching material (15% or 22% as opposed to the standard 10% carbamide peroxide) should not be used. If sensitivity persists, bleaching can be limited to two hours every second day rather than every day. This extends the treatment time but usually controls the sensitivity. In all such cases perseverance is the key to success.

Soft tissue discomfort
There have been some reports of mild tingling sensations in the gums. This usually passes off after a few days. Stopping bleaching will result in a rapid improvement in the situation. When the symptoms have subsided, bleaching can usually be resumed. If the symptoms return, bleaching should be stopped and the dentist contacted for advice. In such circumstances bleaching can usually be completed but it may take significantly longer than anticipated.

What about Chair-side Bleaching?
Chair-side bleaching, sometimes called "power bleaching" or "in-surgery bleaching", is done by the dentist in the surgery using a much higher concentration of hydrogen peroxide (10 times higher than that used for nightguard vital bleaching). This is sometimes combined with the use of light, heat or a laser to try to speed up the reaction of the bleaching gel. However, there is little scientific evidence that the use of lights, heat or lasers improves the outcome of bleaching although the use of such devices may speed up the process.

A chair-side bleaching session may take 90 minutes or longer to complete. A number of these sessions may be required to get a result as good as that achievable with nightguard vital bleaching.

Other Methods of Treating Tooth Discolouration

Should bleaching not produce a satisfactory result, there are other methods of treating discoloured teeth. However, it should be borne in mind that some of the procedures listed below are destructive of tooth tissue and usually more costly than bleaching.

Microabrasion

This involves the use of a mixture of acid and an abrasive material to remove a very small amount of the superficial enamel. In some cases microabrasion can help lighten teeth. This technique, however, is only effective in the treatment of surface stain and discolouration. It does not help in the management of deeper discolouration within the body of the teeth.

Composite

Composite is a tooth-coloured material which can be bonded (glued) to tooth tissue to change the colour and shape of the tooth. A "mock-up" can be done to see if the effect is acceptable before doing it for real. This is a non-destructive approach and involves minimal destruction of enamel.

Porcelain Veneers

Porcelain veneers are thin facings of tooth-coloured porcelain which are glued with composite resin on to the front of the teeth with the aim of improving the appearance. The provision of a veneer may involve the removal of a significant amount of enamel from the front surface of a tooth.

Crowns

Unsightly teeth can be crowned (or capped). Preparation for a crown involves removing all the enamel and a considerable amount of dentine. The tooth is significantly weakened by this process and in one in six teeth crowned the nerve dies as a consequence of this procedure.

Extraction

The tooth can be extracted and replaced in a variety of ways. This approach is very radical and is rarely indicated just for aesthetic reasons.

Chapter 9
Complications and Contraindications

Aim

The aim of this chapter is to discuss the common complications together with the contraindications in undertaking dental bleaching.

Outcome

The practitioner will be familiar with how best to manage or, where possible, avoid problems which may be commonly encountered with bleaching.

Overbleaching

There may be a problem of overbleaching with inside/outside bleaching because it is so effective. Overbleaching may, in part, be associated with the limited amount of dentine remaining within the root-filled tooth. The removal of dentine in accessing the root canal system can be considerable, especially if a high-speed rotary instrument is used within the pulp chamber while attempting to identify a canal opening (Fig 9-1). Unnecessary removal of sound tooth tissue is all too easy when using a high-speed cutting instrument.

Lack of knowledge of the anatomy of the pulp chamber when undertaking endodontic procedures may lead to unnecessary weakening of the tooth. It is very important to remove all the blood breakdown products from the pulp chamber, including the pulp horns, down to a level below the cervical margin. Instead of using a high-speed cutting instrument to complete this procedure, it is much more sensible to use a fine ultrasonic tip for this purpose. Once access has been gained to the pulp chamber the ultrasonic tip can be used to loosen, fragment and flush away the discoloured contents of the coronal pulp space (Fig 9-2).

While overbleaching usually "rebounds" quite quickly, the visual effect can generally be modified by using a relatively dark shade of restorative material to restore the access cavity. To test the visual effect of the selected shade of restorative material, the pulp chamber is filled with water prior to trial insertion of the material. Once the effect has been observed, the material is quickly

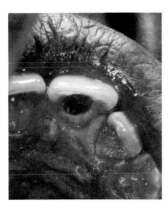

Fig 9-1 Excessive removal of tooth tissue in gaining access. Note the dark stained material still left within the tooth chamber.

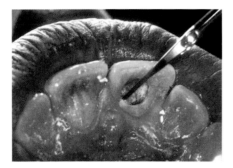

Fig 9-2 Ultrasonic tip cleaning coronal pulp space.

removed using an ultrasonic tip. The material must be removed completely before there is a possibility of polymerisation under ambient operating light. The empty pulp chamber is then dried, etched and primed, with the selected material then being placed according to the manufacturer's directions.

As an alternative to this, the adjacent teeth can be bleached to match the overbleached teeth using conventional nightguard vital bleaching (Figs 9-3 to 9-6).

Wrong Order of Bleaching

It is recommended to bleach especially dark teeth first to match the adjacent teeth before proceeding to bleach the rest of the teeth. This is preferable to bleaching all the teeth first and then trying to bleach the darker teeth to match the newly lighter ones. It is generally difficult to bleach very dark teeth to the brightness of electively lightened adjacent teeth (Figs 9-7 and 9-8).

114

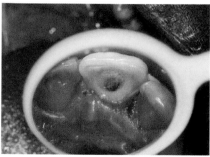

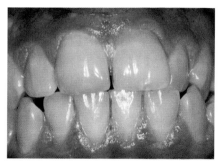

Fig 9-3 Palatal view of the upper left central incisor after bleaching.

Fig 9-4 Labial view of the upper left central incisor before bleaching.

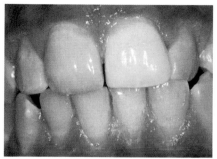

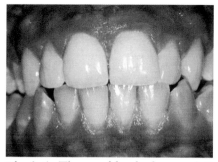

Fig 9-5 Labial view of overbleached upper left central incisor.

Fig 9-6 The overbleached upper left central incisor has been restored and the adjacent teeth bleached to match with nightguard vital bleaching.

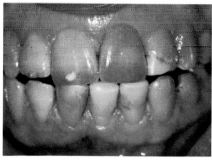

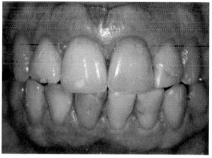

Fig 9-7 Discoloured upper left central incisor adjacent to an upper left lateral incisor restored with a composite tip.

Fig 9-8 The upper left central incisor was bleached first, followed by general bleaching.

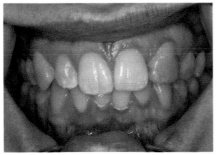

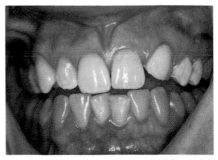

Fig 9-9 Upper left canine in the position of the upper left lateral incisor with a dark shade of composite applied to simulate the appearance of a lateral incisor.

Fig 9-10 Composite removed from the upper left canine to facilitate subsequent bleaching using nightguard vital bleaching.

Bleaching of Teeth Restored with Composite

Composite restorations will not change colour with bleaching. If it is planned to bleach a composite veneered tooth, the veneering composite should, wherever possible, be removed first. This should include the resin tags in the enamel to allow the hydrogen peroxide to penetrate and bleach the discoloured tooth tissue. The teeth should be checked by etching them with phosphoric acid and then by washing and drying them. Any areas that do not appear "frosty" still have resin tags present, which may stop effective bleaching in that area (see Figs 9-9 and 9-10).

If bleached teeth are very light, it may be necessary to use bleach-coloured composites to replace existing restorations. These composites are produced by a number of manufacturers. The main problem with bleach-coloured composites is that they are often opaque white and lack natural translucency. In contrast, regular light-coloured composites are translucent and allow too much light to pass through the bleached tooth, making restoration margins very obvious. Layering techniques will normally overcome this problem. A relatively dark shade of composite is placed initially, followed by progressively lighter shades of composite as the restoration is built outwards towards the front of the restoration (Fig 9-11).

Inappropriate Timing of the Placement of Restorations

It is prudent to complete bleaching to the patient's satisfaction before restoring adjacent teeth or replacing any existing restorations in the bleached

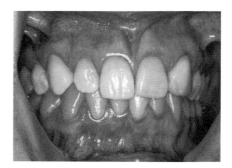

Fig 9-11 Upper left canine recontoured with bleach-coloured composite to better match the colour of the upper left central incisor.

teeth. This is especially important if significant technical costs will be incurred in the provision of porcelain veneers, crowns, implant-retained crowns or bridges.

In the case illustrated (Figs 9-12 to 9-14) two implant-retained crowns were placed without the patient first being asked if she was happy with the colour of her other teeth. Once the implant-retained crowns had been fitted, the patient requested bleaching of the dead root-filled upper right central incisor.

Bleaching was subsequently undertaken using the inside/outside bleaching technique but the patient failed to attend at the appropriate time and continued bleaching beyond the appropriate lightening. The result was to make the implant-retained crowns look too dark.

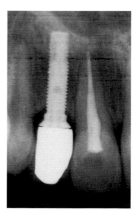

Fig 9-12 Radiograph of root-filled upper right central incisor adjacent to upper right lateral incisor which has been restored with an implant-retained crown.

117

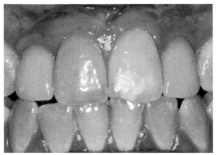

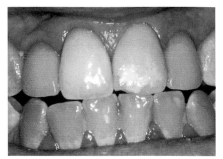

Fig 9-13 Discoloured dead upper right central incisor. Implant-retained crowns at upper right and left lateral incisors.

Fig 9-14 Appearance following overbleaching of the upper right central incisor. Note colour mismatch of implant-retained crowns.

The unfavourable outcome and the costs incurred in replacing the crowns could have been avoided by dealing with any bleaching requirements prior to providing the implant-retained restorations. It is prudent to ask all patients before taking the final shade for a restoration if they are happy with the existing colour of their teeth. If they are not, it is sensible and best practice to complete the bleaching, wait for an appropriate period of time to allow the shade to stabilise, and then proceed to complete any planned restorations.

Failure to Recognise Restorations

Following bleaching, composite restorations can look darker than the lightened teeth. If the dentist fails to note the presence of any existing composite restorations and, as a consequence, omits to warn the patient of the likelihood of a mismatch in colour, the outcome can be a very unhappy patient. Some patients have insisted that these restorations be replaced at no charge to themselves (Fig 9-15).

Dark restorations can often be resurfaced with a lighter material. It is possible to gauge the visual effect of this by removing the surface and sculpting some composite over the restoration. If the appearance is acceptable, resurfacing can be undertaken according to the relevant manufacturer's directions. If the effect is unsatisfactory, the offending restorations will need to be replaced, with the inevitable loss of some sound tooth tissue and enlargement of the preparation.

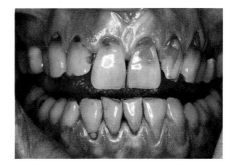

Fig 9-15 Patient with multiple cervical restorations presenting for bleaching. Bleaching is likely to cause marked sensitivity and the restorations will probably require resurfacing, if not replacement, to complete the case.

Very Dark Teeth

Very dark teeth are extremely difficult to bleach. These include teeth seriously darkened by prolonged or repeated exposure to tetracyclines during tooth development. Tetracycline orthophosphate is a very stable compound found in the dentine of tetracycline discoloured teeth. The discolouration caused by this is very difficult to completely eliminate (Fig 9-16).

Less severe yellow/brown tetracycline discolouration is somewhat easier to manage than a dark band of discolouration especially if this is present in the cervical region of the teeth. The visual problem is caused by there being very little enamel in the cervical region to mask the underlying tetracycline discolouration. Bleaching of the teeth will often highlight the dark cervical area. It is important to have reservoirs in the tray over dark or banded areas. An appropriate technique is described in more detail in Chapter 4.

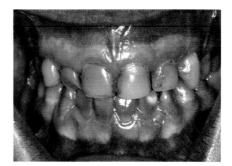

Fig 9-16 Blue/grey tetracycline discolouration. The translucent composite applied on the upper teeth does not conceal the discolouration.

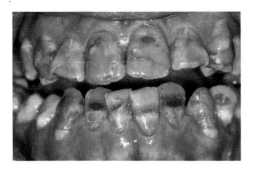

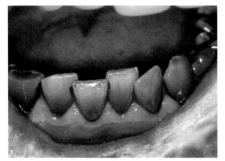

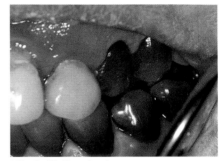

Fig 9-17 Banded tetracycline discolouration in a patient with amelogenesis imperfecta.

Fig 9-18 Porphyria. These teeth will not bleach.

Fig 9-19 Porphyria.

Fig 9-17 shows an example of the effects of banded tetracycline discolouration in a patient with amelogenesis imperfecta. Figs 9-18 and 9-19 show porphyria. These teeth will not bleach.

"Retchers"

Patients with an accentuated gag reflex may find it difficult to wear a bleaching tray. If the tray covers only the anterior teeth, some "retchers" may be able to tolerate nightguard vital bleaching. Using a lower tray to take an upper impression may be one way around the dilemma of obtaining impressions in such patients. Alternatively, acupuncture (the "Fiske" point) may help. In some circumstances it may be appropriate to encourage the patient to have three to four units of alcohol prior to the appointment for impressions. Needless to say, such patients must be told not to drink and drive and should not return to work or operate machinery. The tray will need to be made of a thin material and should not be overextended. Non-compliance in wearing the tray will render the bleaching ineffective.

Retchers unable to tolerate impressions or having a tray in place for several hours at a time may be better treated by means of in-surgery bleaching. However, some of these patients may not be able to tolerate having rubber dam applied for the necessary period of time. In this case, it may be necessary to resort to over-the-counter bleaching strips or some other product not involving the use of a tray or rubber dam. The clinical outcome may have to be a compromise between the patient's wishes and what can actually be achieved.

Body Dysmorphic Disorder

Body dysmorphic disorder, also known as dysmorphophobia, is a severe psychiatric disorder. Patients become obsessed about an imaginary ugliness of part of their body. If the obsession centres on their teeth they may complain that their teeth look too dark, despite objective evidence by reference to a shade guide or colourimeter that this is not the case. Such patients often have a type of obsessive compulsive disorder in which they continually want to bleach their teeth. If bleaching is denied them, they will sometimes get others to obtain bleaching gel from an unsuspecting dentist.

The availability of over-the-counter products and of conventional bleaching products through the internet means that dentally dysmorphophobic patients can readily bypass their dentist and overbleach their teeth. The real dental difficulty with these patients occurs when trying to match new restorations to excessively bleached teeth. The problem is not helped by some enthusiasts of bleaching actively promoting lightening of teeth "beyond the shade B1".

Dysmorphophobic patients with white fluorotic flecks (secondary flecking) need to be treated with caution. Such patients may insist on having their white-flecked teeth overbleached and then treated by means of microabrasion. Remaining unhappy with such treatment, they sometimes insist on having ultrawhite porcelain veneers which, in turn, may still fail to satisfy them (Figs 9-20 and 9-21).

Xerostomia

The lack of saliva in patients with xerostomia could be considered to limit the rate of degradation of peroxide by salivary catalase and peroxidases, and, as a consequence, to be a contraindication to bleaching. On the basis of a study which found no difference in the clearance of peroxide from the oral

121

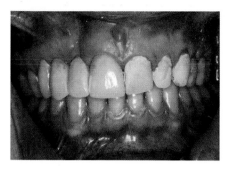

Fig 9-20 History of overbleaching and multiple replacement restorations, culminating in ultrawhite bridgework.

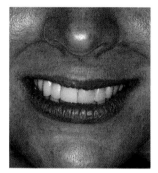

Fig 9-21 Porcelain veneers removed prior to bleaching and re-veneering with bleach-coloured composite.

cavity when comparing adults with normal salivary flow and adults with diminished salivary flow (Sjögren's syndrome), dry mouth, unless very severe, is not in fact a contraindication to bleaching.

Further Reading

Cororve MB, Gleaves DH. Body dysmorphic disorder: a review of conceptualization, assessment and treatment strategies. Clin Psychol Rev 2001;21:949–970.

Hasan JS. Psychological issues in cosmetic surgery: a functional overview. Ann Past Surg 2000;44:89–96.

Marshall MV, Gragg PP, Packman EW et al. Hydrogen peroxide decomposition in the oral cavity. Am J Dent 2001;14:39–45.

Ritvo EC, Melnick I, Marcus GR, Glick ID. Psychiatric conditions in cosmetic surgery patients 2006;22:194–197.

Index

Quintessentials for General Dental Practitioners Series

in 50 volumes

Editor-in-Chief: Professor Nairn H F Wilson

The Quintessentials for General Dental Practitioners Series covers basic principles and key issues in all aspects of modern dental medicine. Each book can be read as a stand-alone volume or in conjunction with other books in the series.

Publication date, approximately

Clinical Practice, Editor: Nairn Wilson

Culturally Sensitive Oral Healthcare	available
Dental Erosion	available
Special Care Dentistry	available
Evidence Based Dentistry	Autumn 2007
Infection Control for the Dental Team	Winter 2007
Therapeutics and Medical Emergencies in the Everyday Clinical Practice of Dentistry	Winter 2007

Oral Surgery and Oral Medicine, Editor: John G Meechan

Practical Dental Local Anaesthesia	available
Practical Oral Medicine	available
Practical Conscious Sedation	available
Minor Oral Surgery in Dental Practice	available

Imaging, Editor: Keith Horner

Interpreting Dental Radiographs	available
Panoramic Radiology	available
21st Century Dental Imaging	available

Periodontology, Editor: Iain L C Chapple

Understanding Periodontal Diseases: Assessment and Diagnostic Procedures in Practice	available
Decision-Making for the Periodontal Team	available
Successful Periodontal Therapy – A Non-Surgical Approach	available
Periodontal Management of Children, Adolescents and Young Adults	available
Periodontal Medicine: A Window on the Body	available
Contemporary Periodontal Surgery – An Illustrated Guide to the Art Behind the Science	Autumn 2007

Endodontics, Editor: John M Whitworth

Rational Root Canal Treatment in Practice	available
Managing Endodontic Failure in Practice	available
Adhesive Restoration of Endodontically Treated Teeth	available

Prosthodontics, Editor: P Finbarr Allen

Teeth for Life for Older Adults	available
Complete Dentures – from Planning to Problem Solving	available
Removable Partial Dentures	available
Fixed Prosthodontics in Dental Practice	available
Occlusion: A Theoretical and Team Approach	Autumn 2007
Managing Orofacial Pain in Practice	Winter 2007

Operative Dentistry, Editor: Paul A Brunton

Decision-Making in Operative Dentistry	available
Aesthetic Dentistry	available
Communicating in Dental Practice	available
Indirect Restorations	available
Dental Bleaching	available
Choosing and Using Dental Materials	Autumn 2007
Composite Restorations in Posterior Teeth	Winter 2007

Paediatric Dentistry/Orthodontics, Editor: Marie Therese Hosey

Child Taming: How to Manage Children in Dental Practice	available
Paediatric Cariology	available
Treatment Planning for the Developing Dentition	available
Managing Dental Trauma in Practice	available

General Dentistry and Practice Management, Editor: Raj Rattan

The Business of Dentistry	available
Risk Management in General Dental Practice	available
Quality Matters: From Clinical Care to Customer Service	available
Practice Management for the Dental Team	Winter 2007

Dental Team, Editor: Mabel Slater

Team Players in Dentistry	Winter 2007

Implantology, Editor: Lloyd J Searson

Implantology in General Dental Practice	available

Quintessence Publishing Co. Ltd., London